Diagnostic History and Physical Examination in Medicine

Paul D. Chan, M.D.

Peter J. Winkle, M.D.

Preface

Diagnostic History & Physical Exam provides a link between the current medical literature and the hospital wards. For each disease covered, the relevant history and physical examination points are listed. Both the pertinent positive and pertinent negative findings are summarized, followed by a complete differential diagnosis. This reference provides help for physicians and medical students who would like to provide comprehensive and analytical patient evaluations; it prevents omission of important history and physical exam findings. **Diagnostic History and Physical Exam** is written in a concise, quickly readable format which is useful to both the clinical student and the experienced physician.

This manual is designed to be used in conjunction with the **Current Clinical Strategies**, medical therapeutics series.

Publishing information for authors may be obtained by writing to:

Current Clinical Strategies Publishing
9550 Warner Ave, Suite 213
Fountain Valley, Ca 92708-2822
Phone: 714-965-9400
FAX: 714-965-9401
e-Mail: 102044.2455@compuserve.com

Printed in USA   ISBN 0-9626030-8-2

CONTENTS

HISTORY & PHYSICAL EXAMINATION

HISTORY

<u>**Identifying Data:**</u> Patient's name; age, race, sex; referring physician or clinic medical record number. Name and reliability of informant (patient, relative).

<u>**Chief Compliant:**</u> Reason given by patient for seeking medical care; place in "quotation marks."

<u>**History of Present Illness (HPI):**</u> Describe the course of the patient's illness, including when it began, character of the symptoms; location where the symptoms began; aggravating or alleviating factors; pertinent positives and negatives, other related diseases; past illnesses or surgeries; past diagnostic testing.

<u>**Past Medical History (PMH):**</u> Past diseases, surgeries, hospitalizations; significant medical problems; history of diabetes, hypertension, peptic ulcer disease, asthma, chronic obstructive pulmonary disease, myocardial infarction, cancer, tuberculosis. In children include birth history, prenatal history, immunizations, type of feedings.

<u>**Medications:**</u>

<u>**Allergies:**</u> Penicillin?

<u>**Family History:**</u> Medical problems in family; specifically ask about problems similar to patient's illness. Asthma, myocardial infraction, heart failure, hypertension, cancer, tuberculosis, diabetes, kidney diseases.

<u>**Social History:**</u> Alcohol, smoking, drug usage. Marital status, children, employment and home situation; exposure to carcinogens or environmental agents. Level of education.

<u>**Review of Systems (ROS):**</u>

General: Weight gain or loss, appetite loss, fever, chills, fatigue, night sweats.

Skin: Rashes, bruising, skin discolorations.

Head: Headaches, dizziness, lumps or masses; seizures, head trauma.

Eyes: Visual changes, visual acuity, visual field deficits.

Ears: Tinnitus, vertigo, pain, hearing loss.

Nose: Nose bleeds, discharge, sinus diseases.

Mouth & Throat: Dental disease, hoarseness, throat pain.

Respiratory: Cough, shortness of breath, sputum (color, amount); history of tuberculosis; vaccination for influenza or pneumococcus.

Cardiovascular: Chest pain, orthopnea, paroxysmal nocturnal dyspnea; dyspnea on exertion, claudication, extremity edema. History of valvular disease, murmur, rheumatic fever.

Gastrointestinal: Odynophagia, dysphagia, abdominal pain, nausea, vomiting, hematemesis, diarrhea, constipation, melena (black tarry stools), hematochezia (bright red blood per rectum), change in appetite.

Genitourinary: Dysuria, change in urine color or character, frequency, hesitancy, hematuria, polyuria, discharge, impotence, testicular masses.

Gynecological: Gravida/para, abortions, last menstrual period (frequency, duration), age of menarche, menopause; dysmenorrhea, contraception, vaginal bleeding; last pelvic exam and pap smear, breast masses, nipple discharge; breast self-examination, mammography.

Endocrine: Polyuria, polydipsia, polyphagia, skin or hair changes, cold or heat intolerance.

Musculoskeletal: Joint pain or swelling, arthritis, myalgias.

Skin and Lymphatics: Easy bruising, bleeding tendencies; lymphadenopathy.

Neuropsychiatric: Weakness, seizures, paresthesias, memory changes, depression.

PHYSICAL EXAMINATION

Vital Signs: Temperature, heart rate, respirations, blood pressure.

Skin: Rashes, scars, moles; capillary refill (in seconds).

Lymph Nodes: Cervical, supraclavicular, axillary, inguina nodes; size, mobility, tenderness, consistency.

Head: Bruising, tenderness, masses. In pediatric patients check fontanels.

Eyes: Pupils equal round and react to light and accommodation (PERRLA); extra ocular movements intact (EOMI); visual fields and acuity. Fundoscopy (fundi, papilledema, arteriovenous nicking, hemorrhages, or exudates); conjunctiva; scleral icterus, ptosis (drooping lid).

Ears: Acuity, tympanic membranes (dull, shiny, intact, injected, bulging).

Nose: Discharge, exudates, nasal flaring.

Mouth & Throat: Mucus membrane color and moisture level; oral lesions, dentition, tonsils.

Neck: Jugular venous distention (JVD), thyromegaly, lymphadenopathy; range of motion, masses, bruits, abdominojugular reflux.

Chest: Equal expansion, tactile fremitus, percussion, auscultation, rhonchi, crackles, rubs, breath sounds, egophony, whispered pectoriloquy.

Heart: Point of maximal impulse (PMI), thrills (palpable turbulence); regular rate and rhythm (RRR), first and second heart sounds (S1 & S2); gallops (S3,

S4), murmurs (grade 1-6), pulses (graded 0-2+).

Breast: Dimpling, tenderness, lumps, nipple discharge, gynecomastia.

Abdomen: Contour (flat, scaphoid, obese, distended); scars, bowel sounds, bruits, tenderness, masses, liver span by percussion; splenomegaly; guarding, rebound, ; percussion note (tympanic), costovertebral angle tenderness (CVAT).

Genitourinary: External lesions, inguinal masses, hernias, scrotum, testicles, varicoceles.

Pelvic Exam: Vaginal mucosa, cervical discharge; uterine size and masses, adnexa, ovaries, suprapubic tenderness.

Extremities: Joint swelling, range of motion, edema (grade 1-4+); cyanosis, clubbing, edema (CCE); pulses (radial, ulnar, femoral, popliteal, posterior tibial, dorsalis pedis; simultaneous palpation of radial and femoral pulses), Homan's sign (dorsiflexion of foot elicits calf tenderness); cyanosis, varicosities.

Rectal Exam: Sphincter tone, masses, hemorrhoids, fissures; test for occult blood; stool in rectal vault, prostate (nodules, tenderness, size).

Neurological: Mental status and affect; cranial nerves 2-12; gait, strength (graded 0-5); touch sensation, pressure, pain, position and vibration; deep tendon reflexes (biceps, triceps, patellar, ankle) (graded 0-4+); Romberg's test (ability of patient to stand erect with arms outstretched and eyes closed).

Cranial Nerve Examination:

   I: Smell

   II: Vision and visual fields;

   III, IV, VI: Pupil responses to light; eye movements, ptosis.

   V: Facial sensation, ability to open jaw against resistance, corneal reflex.

   VII: Close eyes tightly, smile, show teeth.

   VIII: Hearing of watch tic; Weber test (lateralization of sound when tuning fork is placed on top of head); Rinne test (air conduction last longer than bone conduction when tuning fork is placed on mastoid process).

   IX, X: Palette moves in midline when patient says "ah," speech.

   XI: Shoulder shrug and turns head against resistance.

   XII: Stick out tongue in midline. Heal to skin test.

Labs: Electrolytes (sodium, potassium, bicarbonate, chloride, BUN, creatinine), CBC (hemoglobin, hematocrit, WBC count, platelets, differential); x-rays, ECG, urine analysis (UA), liver function test (LFT's).

Assessment (Impression): Assign a number to each problem and discuss separately. Discuss differential diagnosis and support working diagnosis with reasons for excluding other diagnoses.

Plan: Describe therapeutic plan for each numbered problem including testing, laboratory studies, medications, antibiotics.

PROBLEM-ORIENTED DAILY PROGRESS NOTE

Problem List: List each problem separately (heart failure, pneumonia, hypokalemia). Address each problem daily in progress note. Give post-operative day number, antibiotic day number if applicable.

Subjective: Describe how the patient feels in the patient's own words; and give observations about the patient.

Objective: Vital signs, physical exam for each system, laboratory data.

Assessment: Evaluate each numbered problem separately, and discuss the progress of each problem.

Plan: For each numbered problem, discuss any additional orders, changes in drug regimen or plans for discharge or transfer. Discuss conclusions of consultants.

DISCHARGE SUMMARY

Patient's Name and Medical Record Number:

Date of Admission:

Date of Discharge:

Admitting Diagnosis:

Discharge Diagnosis:

Attending or Ward Team Responsible for Patient:

Procedures:

Surgical Procedures, Diagnostic Tests, Invasive Procedures:

Brief History, Pertinent Physical Examination and Laboratory Data: Describe the course of the patient's disease up until the patient came to the hospital including physical exam and laboratory data.

Hospital Course: Describe the course of the patient's illness while in the hospital, including evaluation, treatment, outcome of treatment, and medications given while in the hospital.

Discharged Condition: Describe improvement or deterioration in patient's condition.

Disposition: Describe the situation to which the patient will be discharged (home, nursing home). Indicate who will take care of patient.

Discharged Medications: List medications and instructions for patient on taking the medications.

Discharged Instructions & Follow-up Care: Date of return for follow-up care at clinic; diet, exercise.

Problem List: List all active and past problems.

Copies: Send copies to attending, clinic, consultants.

CARDIOLOGY

CHEST PAIN & MYOCARDIAL INFARCTION

History: Duration of chest pain in hours. Location, radiation, character, intensity, rate of onset (gradual or sudden); relationship to activity; relief by nitroglycerine, rest, antacids; increased in frequency or severity of anginal pattern. Improvement or worsening of pain; occurrence during rest or sleep.

Associated Symptoms: Diaphoresis, nausea, vomiting, dyspnea at rest or on exertion, orthopnea, edema, weakness, palpitations, hemoptysis, dysphagia, cough, sputum, paresthesias of arm, hand, face; syncope.

Aggravating & Relieving Factors: Effect of inspiration, cough or position (supine, upright) on pain; exacerbation by arm, chest or neck movement; effect of eating, aspirin, NSAIDS, alcohol, exertion, anxiety, drinking of cold liquids (esophageal). Cocaine or nicotine patch use.

Cardiac Testing: Past stress testing, angiograms, nuclear scans, ECG's.

Risk Factors: Family history of coronary artery disease before age 55, diabetes, hypertension, smoking, hypercholesterolemia.

PMH: History of diabetes, claudication, stroke. Exercise tolerance; history of peptic ulcer disease, melena, abdominal pain, bleeding risk factors, peripheral vascular disease, pre or post menopausal. Prior history of myocardial infarction, coronary bypass grafting or angioplasty, gastrointestinal bleeding, cerebral vascular bleed (contraindications for thrombolytics).

Physical Exam:

General: Visible pain, apprehension, distress, pallor.

Vitals P (tachycardia), BP in both arms, R (tachypnea), T.

Skin: Cold extremities (peripheral vascular disease), xanthomas (hypercholesterolemia).

HEENT: Fundi, "silver wire" arteries, arteriolar narrowing, A-V nicking, hypertensive retinopathy; carotid pulse amplitude, duration; carotid bruits; jugular venous distention.

Chest: Crackles, percussion note, friction rub.

Heart: Chest wall tenderness (reproduction of pain by palpation), dyskinetic cardiac impulse. Levine's sign (patient describes pain with clenched fist over sternum). Decreased intensity of first heart sound (S1) (LV dysfunction); third heart sound (S3) (heart failure, dilation), S4 gallop (in the left lateral position;

decreased LV compliance due to ischemia); mitral insufficiency murmurer (papillary muscle dysfunction), rub (pericarditis).

Abdomen: Epigastric tenderness (peptic ulcer), hepatomegaly, ascites, pulsatile mass (aortic aneurysm).

Rectal: Occult blood.

Extremities: Edema, femoral bruits, unequal or diminished pulses (aortic dissection); calf pain, swelling (thrombosis).

Labs: ECG: ST segment elevation ≥ 0.1 mV in one or more limb leads, T-wave inversion; Q-wave development. Compare with previous ECG's if available.

CXR: Cardiomegaly, pulmonary edema (CHF).

CPK with MB fraction q8h x 3, LDH, Mg, CBC, electrolytes; echocardiogram

Differential Diagnosis: Myocardial ischemia, peptic ulcer, gastritis, esophageal reflux or rupture, aortic dissection, pericarditis, pulmonary embolism, pleuritis, mitral valve prolapse, pulmonary hypertension, pneumothorax, chest wall pain, Tietze's syndrome (Costochondritis), osteoarthritis (spine, shoulder), mastitis, pancreatitis, cholecystitis, pneumonia, malignancy, breast disease, intercostal neuritis (Zoster), psychogenic.

DYSPNEA

History: Rate of onset of shortness of breath (gradual, sudden), orthopnea (shortness of breath when supine), paroxysmal nocturnal dyspnea (PND). Affect of physical exertion; history of myocardial infarction, syncope. Past episodes of dyspnea; aggravating or relieving factors. Edema, weight gain, lightheadedness, cough, sputum, fever, nausea, fatigue, anxiety.

Past Medical History: Bronchitis, emphysema, heart failure, hypertension, occupational exposures, HIV risk factors, history of asthma.

Medications: Bronchodilators, cardiac medications (noncompliance), drug allergies.

Past Treatment or Testing: Cardiac testing, x-rays, ECG's, spirometry.

Physical Exam:

General: Apprehension, respiratory distress. Fluid input and output balance.

Vitals: BP (supine and upright), P (tachycardia), T, R (tachypnea).

HEENT: Central cyanosis (blue tongue and mucous membranes); jugular venous distention at 45 degrees, carotid pulse, bruits; tracheal deviation (pneumothorax).

Chest: Stridor (foreign body), retractions, breath sounds, wheezing, crackles (rales), rhonchi; dullness to percussion (pleural effusion), barrel chest; unilateral hyperresonance (pneumothorax).

Heart: Lateral displacement of point of maximal impulse, atrial fibrillation (irregular, irregular); S3 gallop (LV dilation), S4 (myocardial infarction and increased myocardial compliance), holosystolic apex murmur (mitral regurgitation); faint heart sounds (pericardial effusion).

Abdomen: Abdominojugular reflux (pressing on abdomen produces increased jugular vein distention), hepatomegaly, liver tenderness.

Extremities: Edema, pulses, cyanosis, clubbing, jaundice.

Labs: ABG, cardiac enzymes; CXR (cardiomegaly, hyperinflation with flattened diaphragms, infiltrates, effusions, Kerley B lines). Spirometry (pre/post bronchodilators).

Electrocardiogram:

    A. ST segment depression or elevation, Q waves, or new left bundle-branch block.

    B. ST elevations in two contiguous leads, with ST depressions in reciprocal leads, are strong predictors of MI and the need for thrombolysis. The earliest signs of transmural injury are hyperacute T waves; Q waves occur later.

Echocardiography: Localized area hypokinesia indicates possible coronary thrombosis; may reveal aortic dissection, mitral valve prolapse, pericardial fluid.

Differential Diagnoses: Heart failure, myocardial infarction, upper airway obstruction, pneumonia, pulmonary edema, sarcoidosis, pulmonary embolism, chronic obstructive pulmonary disease, asthma, pneumothorax, aspiration of foreign body or gastric contents, respiratory muscle disease, kyphoscoliosis, hyperventilation, malignancy, anemia.

EDEMA

History: Duration of edema; localized or generalized; associated pain, redness. History of heart failure, liver, or renal disease; weight changes, shortness of breath, malnutrition, chronic diarrhea (protein losing enteropathy), thyroid disease, pregnancy, estrogens, steroids, vasodilators. Exacerbation by menses, position; allergies to food or substances.

Past Treating and Testing: Cardiac testing, chest x-rays. History of deep vein thrombosis, venous insufficiency, varicose veins. Recent fluid input and output balance.

Meds: Cardiac drugs, furosemide, diuretics, calcium channel blockers.

Physical Exam:

Vitals: BP (orthostatic), P, T, R.

HEENT: Jugular venous distention at 45°; carotid pulse, amplitude, duration.

Chest: Breath sounds, crackles, wheeze, dullness to percussion.

Heart: Displacement of point of maximal impulse, atrial fibrillation (irregular, irregular); S3 gallop (LV dilation), rubs.

Abdomen: Abdominojugular reflux, ascites, hepatomegaly, splenomegaly, distention, fluid wave, shifting dullness.

Extremities: Pitting or non-pitting edema, varicose veins, redness, warmth; mottled, brown discoloration of ankle skin (venous insufficiency); leg circumference, tenderness, Homan's sign (dorsiflexion elicits pain; thrombosis); pulses, cyanosis, clubbing.

Differential Diagnosis:

Unilateral Edema: Venous obstruction (DVT, thrombophlebitis); lymphatic obstruction (neoplasm - pelvic, lymphoma).

Generalized Edema: Renal (acute glomerulonephritis, nephrotic syndrome, renal failure), cardiac (CHF), liver disease (cirrhosis, obstruction of hepatic venous outflow), vascular disease (AV fistula, obstruction of inferior or superior vena cava).

Endocrine: Thyroid hormone, mineralocorticoid excess, hypoalbuminemia (protein losing enteropathy, malnutrition).

Miscellaneous: Chronic anemia, angioedema (hereditary/acquired), iatrogenic edema.

CONGESTIVE HEART FAILURE

History: Duration of dyspnea; gradual or sudden onset; paroxysmal nocturnal dyspnea (PND), orthopnea; number of pillows needed under back when supine to prevent dyspnea; edema of lower extremities, dyspnea on exertion (DOE). Exercise tolerance (present and previously). Weight gain. Patient's subjective opinion of severity of dyspnea compared with past episodes.

Associated Symptoms: Fatigue, chest pain, pleuritic pain, cough, fever, chills, sputum, nausea, vomiting, diaphoresis, palpitations, nocturia, syncope.

Past Medical History: Past episodes of heart failure; hypertension, excess salt or fluid intake; noncompliance with diuretics, digoxin, antihypertensives; alcoholism, drug use, diabetes, coronary artery disease, myocardial infarction, heart murmur, arrhythmias.

Thyroid disease, anemia, pulmonary disease.

Past Testing: Echocardiograms for ejection fraction, cardiac testing, nuclear scans, angiograms, ECG's.

Risk Factors: Smoking, diabetes, family history of coronary artery disease or heart failure, hypercholesterolemia, hypertension.

Precipitating Factors: Infections, noncompliance with low salt diet; excessive fluid intake; anemia, hyperthyroidism, pulmonary embolism, nonsteroidal anti-inflammatory drugs, renal insufficiency; adverse drug reactions (beta blockers, calcium blockers, antiarrhythmics, cocaine).

Treatment in Emergency Room: IV Lasix given, volume diuresed. Recent fluid input and output balance.

Physical Exam:

General: Respiratory distress; anxiety, diaphoresis.

Vitals: BP (hypotension or hypertension), P (tachycardia), T, R (tachypnea).

HEENT: Jugular venous distention (at 45° measure vertical distance from the sternal angle to top of column of blood = jugular venous pressure in cm H_2O); hepatojugular reflux (pressing on abdomen causes jugular venous distention); carotid pulse, amplitude, duration, bruits. Acral cyanosis.

Chest: Breath sounds, crackles, wheeze, rhonchi; dullness to percussion (pleural effusion).

Heart: Lateral displacement of point of maximal impulse; atrial fibrillation (irregular, irregular); S3 gallop (LV dilation), holosystolic apex murmur (mitral regurgitation).

Abdomen: Ascites, hepatomegaly, liver tenderness.

Extremities: Edema, pulses, jaundice, muscle wasting; cool extremities.

Labs: CXR: Cardiomegaly, perihilar congestion; vascular cephalization (increased density of upper lobe vasculature); Kerley B lines (horizontal streaks in lower lobes), pleural effusions.

ECG Left ventricular hypertrophy, ectopic beats, atrial fibrillation. Electrolytes, BUN, creatinine, sodium; CBC; serial cardiac enzymes, CPK, MB, LDH.

Differential Diagnosis of Conditions That Mimic or Provoke Heart Failure:

- Coronary artery disease & myocardial infarction
- Hypertension

- Aortic or mitral valve disease
- Cardiomyopathies: Hypertrophic, idiopathic dilated, postpartum, genetic, toxic, nutritional, metabolic
- Myocarditis: Infectious, toxic, immune
- Pericardial constriction
- Tachyarrhythmias or bradyarrhythmias
- Pulmonary embolism
- Pulmonary disease
- Congenital abnormalities
- High output states: Anemia, hyperthyroidism, A-V fistulas, Paget's disease, fibrous dysplasia, multiple myeloma
- Renal failure, nephrotic syndrome

Factors that Precipitate Heart Failure:

Increase Demand: Anemia, fever, infection, excess dietary salt, renal failure, liver failure, thyrotoxicosis, AV fistula, pregnancy, high altitude. Arrhythmias, cardiac ischemia/infarction, pulmonary emboli, alcohol abuse (thiamine deficiency), uncontrolled hypertension.

Medication Related: Antiarrhythmics (disopyramide), negative inotropic agents (beta-blockers, calcium blockers), steroids, NSAID's, noncompliance, excessive Intravenous fluids

New York Heart Association Classification:

Class I: Symptomatic only with strenuous activity.

Class II: Symptomatic with usual level of activity.

Class III: Symptomatic with minimal activity, but asymptomatic at rest.

Class IV: Symptomatic at rest.

PALPITATIONS & ATRIAL FIBRILLATION

History: Palpitations (rapid or irregular heart beat); dizziness, nausea, dyspnea, edema; duration of atrial fibrillation. Results of previous ECG's.

Associated Symptoms: Chest pain, pleuritic pain, syncope, weakness, fatigue, diaphoresis, symptoms of hyperthyroidism.

Cardiac History: Hypertension, salt intake, coronary disease, rheumatic heart disease, cardiomyopathies, arrhythmias; exercise tolerance.

Underlying Conditions: Pneumonia, diabetes, noncompliance with cardiac medications, pericarditis, hyperthyroidism, pulmonary embolism, pneumothorax, aminophylline, myocardial infarction, electrolyte abnormalities, COPD, mitral valve stenosis, hypokalemia; diet pills, decongestants, alcohol, caffeine, cocaine. Bleeding risk factors (ulcers, ataxia).

Physical Exam:

Vitals: BP (hypotension), P (irregular tachycardia), T, R.

HEENT: Retinal hemorrhages; jugular venous distention; carotid pulse duration, amplitude, bruits; thyromegaly (hyperthyroidism).

Chest: Crackles (rales).

Heart: Irregular, irregular rhythm; dyskinetic apical pulse, displaced point of maximal impulse, S4, murmur (rheumatic fever); pericardial rub (pericarditis). Peripheral pulses with irregular timing and amplitude.

Rectal: Occult blood.

Extremities: Edema, cyanosis, ecchymoses, petechia (emboli). Femoral artery bruits (atherosclerosis).

Neuro: Motor weakness (hemiparesis), CN 2-12, sensory; plantar responses; dysphasia, dysarthria (stroke); tremor (hyperthyroidism).

Labs: Sodium, potassium, BUN, creatinine; magnesium; drug levels; CBC; serial cardiac enzymes; CPK, LDH, Mg. CXR.

ECG: Irregular R-R intervals with no P waves. Ventricular rate is irregularly irregular. Irregular baseline with rapid fibrillary waves (more than 320 per minute). The usual ventricular response rate is 130-180 per minute.

Echocardiogram for atrial chamber size.

Differential Diagnosis of Atrial Fibrillation:

Lone Atrial Fibrillation: No underlying disease state.

Cardiac Causes: Hypertensive heart disease with left ventricular hypertrophy, heart failure, mitral valve stenosis or regurgitation, pericarditis, hypertrophic cardiomyopathy, coronary artery disease, myocardial infarction, atrial septal defect, aortic stenosis, infiltrative diseases (amyloidosis, cardiac tumors).

Noncardiac Causes: Hypoglycemia, theophylline intoxication, acute pulmonary disease (pneumonia, asthma, chronic obstructive pulmonary disease, pulmonary embolus), heavy alcohol intake or alcohol withdrawal, hyperthyroidism, severe acute stress or systemic illness, electrolyte abnormalities. Stimulant abuse, excess tobacco, xanthine (tea), chocolate, over-the-counter cold remedies, street drugs.

HYPERTENSION

History: Degree of blood pressure elevation; patient's baseline BP from records; paroxysmal or sustained hypertension; baseline BUN and creatinine. Age of onset of hypertension.

Associated Symptoms: Chest or back pain (aortic dissection), headaches, dyspnea, orthopnea, dizziness, blurred vision (hypertensive retinopathy); nausea, vomiting, headache (pheochromocytoma); lethargy, confusion (encephalopathy).

Paroxysms of tremor, palpitations, diaphoresis, diarrhea; edema, thyroid disease, heart failure, angina, hematuria; flank pain, dysuria, polyuria, urinary infections (renal disease). Weight gain, alcohol withdrawal. Noncompliance with antihypertensives (clonidine or beta-blocker withdrawal), excessive salt, alcohol.

Medications: Over-the-counter cold remedies, beta agonists, diet pills, eye drops (sympathomimetics), bronchodilators, cocaine, amphetamines, nonsteroidal anti-inflammatory agents, oral contraceptives, adrenal steroids, MAO-inhibitors.

Risk Factors for Coronary Artery Disease: Family history of coronary artery disease before age 55, diabetes, hypertension, smoking, hypercholesterolemia.

Past Testing: Urinalysis, ECG, creatinine.

Family History: Hypertension, renal disease, pheochromocytoma.

Physical Exam:

General: Delirium, confusion, agitation (hypertensive encephalopathy).

Vitals: Supine and upright blood pressure (correct size cuff; 2 readings); BP in all extremities.

HEENT: Hypertensive retinopathy, hemorrhages, exudates, "cotton wool" spots, A-V nicking; papilledema; thyromegaly (hyperthyroidism). Jugular venous distention, wave forms, carotid pulse and bruits.

Chest: Crackles (rales, pulmonary edema), wheeze; intercostal bruits (aortic coarctation)

Heart: Rhythm; laterally displaced, sustained, forceful, apical impulse with patient in left lateral position (ventricular hypertrophy); narrowly split S2 with increased aortic component; systolic ejection murmurs (aorta outflow turbulence).

Abdomen: Renal bruits (systolic and diastolic bruit just below costal margin, renal artery stenosis); abdominal aortic enlargement or pulsations (aortic aneurysm), hepatomegaly, renal masses, enlarged kidney (polycystic renal disease); costovertebral angle tenderness. Truncal obesity (Cushing's syndrome).

Skin: Striae, skin atrophy (Cushing's syndrome), uremic frost (chronic renal failure); hirsutism (adrenal hyperplasia); plethora, (pheochromocytoma).

Extremities: Asymmetric or delayed femoral to radial pulses; simultaneous palpation of femoral and brachial pulses (coarctation of aortic); decreased peripheral pulses; femoral bruits, edema, elevation pallor, dependent rubor, skin atrophy (peripheral vascular disease); tremor (pheochromocytoma, hyperthyroidism).

Neuro: Mental status, rapid return phase of deep tendon reflexes (hyperthyroidism), localized weakness (stroke), cranial nerve palsies, visual acuity.

Labs: Potassium, BUN, creatinine, glucose, calcium, uric acid. CBC, fasting lipid panel. UA with microscopic analysis (RBC casts, hematuria, proteinuria). 24 hour urine for metanephines and plasma catecholamines (pheochromocytoma).

ECG: left ventricular hypertrophy.

CXR: cardiomegaly, indentation of aorta (coarctation), rib notching.

Differential Diagnosis of Hypertension:

A. **Primary (essential) Hypertension (90%)**

B. **Secondary Hypertension:** Renovascular hypertension, pheochromocytoma and cocaine use, withdrawal from alpha2 stimulants, clonidine or beta blockers, or alcohol; and noncompliance with antihypertensive medications; ingestion of a tyramine-containing food while taking a monoamine oxidase inhibitor.

PERICARDITIS

History: Sharp pleuritic chest pain; onset, intensity, radiation. Exacerbated by supine position, coughing or deep inspiration; relieved by leaning forward; referred to trapezius ridge; fever, chills, palpitations.

History of recent upper respiratory infection, autoimmune disease; prior episodes; tuberculosis exposure; intravenous drug abuse, dyspnea; myalgias, arthralgias, rashes, fatigue, anorexia, weight loss, kidney disease.

Medications: Hydralazine, procainamide, isoniazid, penicillin, minoxidil.

Physical Exam:

Vitals: BP, P (tachycardia), T, R; pulsus paradoxus (drop in systolic BP >10 mmHg with inspiration).

HEENT: Cornea, sclera, iris lesions; oral ulcers (lupus); jugular venous distention (cardiac tamponade).

Skin: Malar rash (butterfly rash), discoid rash (lupus).

Chest: Crackles (rales), rhonchi.

Heart: Rhythm; friction rub on end-expiration while sitting forward; cardiac rub with 1-3 components at lower left sternal border; distant heart sounds (pericardial effusion).

Rectal: Occult blood.

Extremities: Arthralgias, arthritis.

Labs: ECG: diffuse, downwardly, concave, ST segment elevation in all 3 standard limb leads and several precordial leads; upright T waves, PR segment depression, low QRS voltage.

CXR: large cardiac silhouette; "water bottle sign"; pericardial calcifications.

Echocardiogram.

Increased WBC; UA, urine protein, RBC's; CPK, MB, LDH, blood culture, increased ESR.

Differential Diagnosis: Idiopathic, infectious (viral, bacterial, mycoplasmal, mycobacterial), Lyme disease, uremia, neoplasm, connective tissue disease, lupus, rheumatic fever, polymyositis, aortic aneurysm (with leak), myxedema, sarcoidosis, post myocardial infarction (Dressler's syndrome), drugs (penicillin, isoniazid, procainamide, hydralazine).

SYNCOPE

History: Time and location where loss of consciousness occurred. Duration of unconsciousness, sudden or gradual onset; observations by witnesses; activity before and after event. Body position, arm position (reaching), and neck position (turning to side); mental status before and after event. Precipitants (fear, tension, hunger, pain).

Seizure activity (tonic/clonic activity). Cough, micturition, defecation, exertion syncope; Valsalva, hyperventilation; chest pain trauma; chest pain, palpitations, tonic-clonic movements headache, collar tightness.

Prodromal Symptoms: Diaphoresis, blurred or dimming vision, nausea, tinnitus, aura (carotid sinus hypersensitivity syndrome).

Symptoms of the Event: Post-syncopal lethargy, confusion, lightheadedness, vertigo, flushing; calf pain, dyspnea, hemoptysis (pulmonary embolism), incontinence of stool/urine, tongue biting.

Rate of return to alertness (delayed or spontaneous), weakness, cyanosis, pallor, melena.

Past Medical History: History of syncope, stroke, transient ischemic attacks, seizures, valvular disease, arrhythmias, hypertension, anemia, diabetes, anxiety attacks, exercise.

Medications Causing Syncope: Antihypertensives (beta blockers, calcium blockers), diuretics, antiarrhythmics, anticonvulsants, sedatives, insulin, oral hypoglycemics, alcohol, phenothiazines, nitrates, CNS depressants, cocaine, diet pills, cold remedies, excess caffeine.

Past Testing: 24 hour Holter, cardiac testing, ECG, EEG.

Physical Exam:

General: Level of alertness.

Vitals: T, R; orthostatic vitals (supine and after standing 2-5 minutes), P.

HEENT: Cranial tenderness, bruising (trauma). Pupil size and reactivity, extraocular movements; tongue or buccal lacerations (seizure); flat jugular veins (volume depletion); carotid pulse amplitude and duration; carotid or vertebral bruits.

Skin: Turgor, capillary refill, pallor.

Chest: Breath sounds, crackles, rhonchi (aspiration).

Heart: Irregular rhythm (atrial fibrillation), S2, S3, S4; systolic ejection murmurs (aortic stenosis), cardiac rub.

Abdomen: Bruits, tenderness pulsatile mass.

Genitourinary/Rectal: Occult blood; urinary or fecal incontinence (seizure).

Extremities: Palpate extremities for trauma.

Neuro: Cranial nerves 2-12, strength, gait, coordination, sensory, memory, tendon reflexes, mental status; nystagmus, facial paralysis. Turn patient's head side to side, up and down; have patient reach above head, bend down and pick up object, resist a push.

Labs: ECG: arrhythmias, Q waves, blocks. CXR, electrolytes, glucose, Mg, BUN, creatinine, CBC; EEG, 24-hour Holter monitor.

Differential Diagnosis:

1. Vasovagal/Vasopressor syncope (simple faint)

2. Cardiac Syncope:
   a. Aortic stenosis, idiopathic hypertrophic subaortic stenosis (IHHS), pulmonic valve stenosis, pulmonary emboli.
   c. Dysrhythmia - Heart block (Adam-Stokes attacks), paroxysmal tachycardia, sinoatrial dysfunction (sick sinus syndrome, sinus arrest), atrial/ventricular dysrhythmias.
3. Vascular Syncope:
   a. Orthostatic Hypotension: Volume depletion (hemorrhage)
   b. Medication related: Diuretics, tricyclic antidepressants, antihypertensives
   c. Neurologic disease: Diabetic neuropathy, tabes dorsalis (neurosyphilis)
4. Cerebrovascular Syncope:
   a. Atherosclerotic disease, thrombus, embolism
   b. Vertebrobasilar arterial insufficiency
   c. Subclavian steal syndrome, aortic arch syndrome
5. Miscellaneous: Carotid sinus syndrome, micturition/cough syncope, hysterical fainting, hypoglycemia, hyperventilation.

PULMONOLOGY

HEMOPTYSIS

History: Quantify blood, acuteness of onset, color (bright red, dark, rusty), character of sputum (food particles, clots); dyspnea, pleuritic chest pain; smoking, fever, chills, past bronchoscopies, exposure to tuberculosis or asbestos; hematuria, weight loss, anorexia, malaise.

Farm exposure; hoarseness, foreign body aspiration, nasal or sinus pain, HIV risk factors (pulmonary Kaposi's sarcoma), leg pain or swelling (pulmonary embolism), valvular disease, bronchitis, pneumonia, COPD, heart failure, anticoagulants, aspirin, NSAID's. Family history of bleeding disorders. Prior chest X-rays, tuberculin testing (PPD).

Physical Exam:

General: Dyspnea, respiratory distress.

Vitals: T, R (tachypnea), P (tachycardia), BP (hypotension); assess hemodynamic status.

HEENT: Sinus tenderness, nasal or oropharyngeal lesions; telangiectasias on lips or buccal mucosa (Rendu-Osler-Weber disease); ulcerations of nasal septum (Wegener's granulomatosis), jugular venous distention; gingival disease.

Lymph Nodes: Cervical, scalene or supraclavicular adenopathy (Virchow's nodes, intrathoracic malignancy).

Chest: Stridor, tenderness or splinting of chest wall; rhonchi, apical crackles (tuberculosis); localized wheezing (foreign body, malignancy); basilar crackles (pulmonary edema), pleural friction rub, breast masses (metastasis).

Heart: Mitral stenosis murmur (diastolic rumble, opening snap), right ventricular gallop; accentuated, loud, second heart sound.

Abdomen: Masses; liver nodules (metastases), tenderness.

Extremities: Petechiae, ecchymoses (coagulopathy); cyanosis, tenderness, calf swelling (pulmonary embolism); clubbing (pulmonary disease or cancer), edema; bone pain (metastasis).

Neuro: Cranial nerve palsies, tremor, weakness.

Rectal: Occult blood.

Skin: Purple plaques (Kaposi's sarcoma); rashes (paraneoplastic syndromes).

Labs: Sputum gram stain, KOH (fungi), cytology, acid fast bacteria stain; CBC, platelets, ABG; pH of expectorated blood (alkaline=pulmonary; acidic=GI);

UA (hematuria); PT/PTT, bleeding time; creatinine, BUN; anti-glomerular basement membrane antibody, antinuclear antibody; PPD, coccidiomycoses skin test, EKG. Chest x-ray. CT scan, bronchoscopy.

Differential Diagnosis:

Infection: Bronchitis, bronchiectasis, pneumonia, lung abscess, tuberculosis, fungal infection.

Neoplasms: Bronchogenic carcinoma, bronchial adenoma, metastatic, Kaposi's sarcoma.

Cardiovascular: Pulmonary infarction, mitral stenosis, pulmonary edema.

Miscellaneous: Trauma, foreign body, bleeding diathesis (epistaxis, oropharyngeal, Goodpasture's syndrome, lupus, idiopathic hemosiderosis, Wegener's granulomatosis.

WHEEZING & ASTHMA

History: Onset, duration and progression of wheezing; dyspnea; patient's subjective opinion of severity of attack; cough, fever, chills, purulent sputum; frequency of exacerbations and hospitalizations; history of steroid dependency, intubation, home oxygen or nebulizer use.

Exposure to allergens (foods, pollen, animals, drugs); activities or seasons that provoke symptoms, occupational exposures; exacerbation by exercise, emotions, aspirin, beta- blockers, new medications, recent upper respiratory infection; chest pain, edema.

Treatment given in emergency room; response to medications.

Past Pulmonary History: Course of previous episodes of asthma; emphysema, bronchitis, pneumonia, smoking. Baseline arterial blood gas results; past pulmonary function testing, skin allergy testing; ill contacts; foreign body aspiration.

Family History: Family history of asthma, allergies, hay-fever, atopic dermatitis. Home dust/pollen control measures.

Physical Exam:

General: Dyspnea, respiratory distress, diaphoresis, somnolence.

Vitals: T, R (tachypnea >28/min), P (tachycardia), BP (widened pulse pressure, hypotension), pulsus paradoxus (inspiratory drop in systolic blood pressure; >10 mmHg = severe attack).

HEENT: Conjunctival injection; nasal flaring, erythema, congestion. Cyanosis, jugular venous distention; stridor, tracheal deviation (pneumothorax).

Chest: Prolonged expiratory wheeze; rhonchi; decreased intensity of breath sounds; accessory muscle use (sternocleidomastoids), barrel chest, increased anteroposterior diameter (hyperinflation), retractions.

Heart: Decreased cardiac dullness to percussion (hyperinflation); third heart sound gallop (S3, cor pulmonale), increased intensity of pulmonic component of second heart sound (P2, pulmonary hypertension).

Abdomen: Retractions, tenderness.

Extremities: Cyanosis, edema, clubbing.

Skin: Atopic dermatitis, urticaria.

Neuro: Decreased mental status, confusion.

Labs: CXR: hyperinflation, bullae, flattening of diaphragms; small, elongated heart.

ABG: respiratory alkalosis, hypoxia.

Sputum gram stain; CBC (eosinophilia), electrolytes, theophylline level.

ECG: sinus tachycardia, right axis deviation, right ventricular hypertrophy. Pulmonary function tests.

Differential Diagnosis: Asthma, bronchitis, emphysema, pneumonia, acute left ventricular heart failure, COPD, anaphylaxis, upper airway obstruction; carcinoid, pulmonary embolism, vasculitis, endobronchial tumors.

CHRONIC OBSTRUCTIVE PULMONARY DISEASE

History: Duration of wheezing; dyspnea, cough, fever, chills; increased sputum production; sputum quantity, consistency, color; smoking (pack-years), occupational exposures, allergies; chest trauma, noncompliance with medications. Patient's subjective opinion of severity of attack. Baseline blood gas from chart.

Associated Symptoms: Chest pain, pleurisy. Adverse drug reactions (NSAIDS, beta blockers, cholinergic agents, sedatives); allergic reaction, smoking.

Past History: Frequency of exacerbations, home oxygen use, steroid dependency, history of intubations, nebulizer use; pneumonia, past pulmonary function tests, "blue bloater" or "pink puffer". Productive cough for at least 3 months of the year for 2 consecutive years (chronic bronchitis). Diabetes, heart failure, family history of emphysema, alcohol abuse.

Treatment given in Emergency Room.

Physical Exam:

General: Cachexia, diaphoresis, respiratory distress; speech interrupted by breaths.

Vitals: T, R (tachypnea), P (tachycardia), BP.

HEENT: Pursed-lip breathing, jugular venous distention. Mucous membrane or perioral cyanosis.

Chest: Barrel chest, retractions, accessory muscle use (sternocleidomastoids), supraclavicular retractions, prolonged expiratory wheezing, rhonchi. Decreased air movement in the chest, hyperinflation.

Heart: Right ventricular heave, S3 gallop (cor pulmonale).

Abdomen: Retractions.

Extremities: Cyanosis, edema, clubbing.

Neuro: Decreased mental status, somnolence, confusion.

Labs: CXR: Diaphragm flattening, bullae, hyperaeration.

ABG: respiratory alkalosis (early), acidosis (late), hypoxia. Sputum gram stain, culture, CBC, electrolytes.

ECG: Sinus tachycardia, right axis deviation, right ventricular hypertrophy, PVC's.

Differential Diagnosis: COPD, emphysema, chronic bronchitis, asthmatic bronchitis, pneumonia, heart failure, alpha-1-antitrypsin deficiency, cystic fibrosis, kyphoscoliosis, obstructive sleep apnea.

PULMONARY EMBOLISM

History: Sudden onset of pleuritic chest pain and dyspnea. Unilateral leg pain, swelling; fever, cough, hemoptysis, diaphoresis, syncope. History of deep vein thrombosis.

Virchow's Triad: Immobility, trauma, hypercoagulability; malignancy (pancreas, lung, genitourinary, stomach, breast, pelvic, bone); estrogens (oral contraceptives), history of heart failure, surgery, obesity, pregnancy.

Physical Exam:

General: Dyspnea, apprehension, diaphoresis.

Vitals: T (fever), R (tachypnea, >16/min), P (tachycardia >100/min), BP (hypotension).

HEENT: Jugular venous distention, prominent jugular A-waves.

Chest: Crackles (rales); tenderness or splinting of chest wall, pleural friction rub; breast mass (malignancy).

Heart: Right ventricular gallop; accentuated, loud, pulmonic component of second heart sound (S2); S3 or S4 gallop; murmur.

Extremities: Cyanosis; calf redness, tenderness, Homan's Sign (pain with dorsiflexion of foot), warmth; swelling, increased calf circumference (>2 cm difference).

Rectal: Occult blood.

Genitourinary: Testicular or pelvic masses.

Neuro: Altered mental status.

Labs: ABG: Hypoxemia, hypocapnia, respiratory alkalosis.

Lung Scan: Ventilation/perfusion mismatch.

Pulmonary angiogram: Arterial filling defects.

CXR: Elevated hemidiaphragm, wedge shaped infiltrate; localized oligemia; effusion, segmental atelectasis.

ECG: Sinus tachycardia, nonspecific ST-T wave changes, QRS changes (acute right shift, S_1Q_3 pattern); right heart strain pattern (P-pulmonale, right bundle branch block, right axis deviation).

Differential Diagnosis: Heart failure, myocardial infarction, upper airway obstruction, pneumonia, pulmonary edema, sarcoidosis, pneumoconioses, pulmonary embolism, respiratory muscle disease, chronic obstructive pulmonary disease, asthma, aspiration of foreign body or gastric contents, hyperventilation.

INFECTIOUS DISEASES

FEVER & SEPSIS

History: Degree of fever; time of onset, pattern of fever; shaking chills (rigors), cough, sputum, sore throat, headache, neck stiffness, dysuria, frequency; night sweats; vaginal discharge, back pain; myalgias, nausea, vomiting, diarrhea, malaise, anorexia.

Chest or abdominal pain, ear, bone or joint pain; recent antipyretic use. Cirrhosis, diabetes, valvular disease, recent surgery; AIDS risk factors, prosthetic implants; central IV lines.

Exposure to tuberculosis or hepatitis; travel history, animal exposure; recent dental GI procedures. Ill contacts; IV or Foley catheter; antibiotic or alcohol use. Recent WBC differential, allergies.

Physical Exam:
General: Lethargy, toxic appearance.

Vitals: Temperature (fever curve), R, P (tachycardia), BP (hypotension).

HEENT: Papilledema; dental infection, tooth tenderness, tympanic membrane inflammation (otitis media), sinus tenderness; pharyngeal erythema; lymphadenopathy, neck rigidity.

Breast: Tenderness, masses.

Chest: Rhonchi, crackles, dullness to percussion (pneumonia).

Heart: Murmurs (endocarditis).

Abdomen: Masses, liver tenderness, hepatomegaly, splenomegaly; Murphy's Sign (right upper quadrant tenderness and arrest of respiration secondary to pain, cholecystitis); shifting dullness, ascites. Costovertebral angle or suprapubic tenderness.

Extremities: Cellulitis, infected decubitus ulcers or wounds; IV catheter tenderness (phlebitis), calf tenderness, Homan's sign; joint tenderness, swelling (septic arthritis). Osler's nodes, Janeway's lesions (peripheral lesions of endocarditis).

Rectal: Prostate tenderness; rectal flocculence, fissures, ulcers.

Pelvic/Genitourinary: Foley catheter; pelvic exam, cervical discharge, cervical motion tenderness; adnexal or uterine tenderness, masses; genital herpes lesions.

Skin: Color, temperature, capillary refill; rash, purpura, petechia (septic emboli, meningococcemia), desquamation (toxic shock syndrome); ecthyma gangrenosum (purpuric necrotic plaque of pseudomonas infection). Pustules, cellulitis, furuncles, abscesses, cysts; malar/discoid rash (lupus).

Labs: CBC, blood C&S x 2, BUN, creatinine, UA, urine C&S; lumbar puncture; blood, urine, sputum, wound cultures; sputum gram stain; tuberculin skin test, CXR; abdomen X-ray; gallium, indium scans.

Differential Diagnosis:

Infectious Causes: Abscesses, mycobacterial infections (tuberculosis), cystitis, pyelonephritis, endocarditis, wound infection, diverticulitis, cholangitis, osteomyelitis, IV catheter phlebitis, sinusitis, otitis media, upper respiratory infection, pharyngitis, pelvic infection, cellulitis, hepatitis, infected decubitus ulcer, furuncle, peritonitis, abdominal abscess, perirectal abscess, AIDS, mastitis; viral, parasite infections.

Malignancies: Lymphomas, leukemia, solid tumors or carcinomas.

Connective Tissue Diseases: Lupus, rheumatic fever, rheumatoid arthritis, temporal arteritis, sarcoidosis, polymyalgia rheumatica.

Other Causes of Fever: Atelectasis, drug fever, pulmonary emboli, pericarditis, pancreatitis, factitious fever, alcohol withdrawal. Deep vein thrombosis, myocardial infarction, gout, porphyria, thyroid storm, Addisonian crisis.

Medications Associated with Fever: Aspirin, barbiturates, H2 blockers, hydralazine, isoniazid, methyldopa, nitrofurantoin, penicillins, phenytoin, procainamide, quinidine, sulfonamides.

COUGH & PNEUMONIA

History: Duration of cough, chills, rigors, fever; rate of onset of symptoms. Sputum color, quantity, consistency, odor, blood (rust colored). Living situation (nursing home or hospital). Recent antibiotic use.

Associated Symptoms: Pleuritic pain, dyspnea, orthopnea, malaise, sore throat, rhinorrhea, headache, stiff neck, ear pain; abdominal pain, nausea, vomiting, diarrhea, myalgias, arthralgias.

Past Pulmonary History: Previous pneumonia, Pneumocystis pneumonia, intravenous drug abuse, AIDS risk factors. Diabetes, heart failure, COPD, asthma, immunosuppression, alcoholism, steroids, chemotherapy; ill contacts, history of aspiration, sedatives; smoking, travel history, exposure to tuberculosis, asbestos. Pneumococcal, influenza vaccination; tuberculin testing.

Physical Exam:

General: Respiratory distress, dehydration.

Vitals: T (fever), R (tachypnea), P (tachycardia), BP.

HEENT: Tympanic membranes, pharyngeal erythema, lymphadenopathy, neck rigidity, meningeal signs.

Chest: Unilateral splinting; dullness to percussion, tactile fremitus (increased vocal conduction; rhonchi; end-inspiratory crackles; bronchial breath sounds with decreased intensity; whispered pectoriloquy, egophony (E to A changes).

Extremities: Cyanosis, clubbing.

Neuro: Gag reflex, mental status.

Labs: CBC, electrolytes, BUN, creatinine, glucose; UA, ECG. ABG.

CXR: segmental consolidation, air bronchograms, atelectasis, effusion.

Sputum Gram stain: >25 WBC per low-power field, bacteria.

Differential Diagnosis: Pneumonia, CHF, asthma, bronchitis, viral infection, pulmonary embolism, pneumonitis, malignancy.

Possible Etiologic Agents of Community Acquired Pneumonia:

Age 5-40 (without underlying lung disease): Viral, mycoplasma pneumoniae, chlamydia pneumoniae (TWAR), streptococcus pneumoniae, legionella.

>40 (no underlying lung disease): Streptococcus pneumonia, group A streptococcus, H. influenza.

>40 (with underlying disease): Klebsiella pneumonia, Enterobacteriaceae, legionella sp., staphylococcus aureus, chlamydia pneumoniae.

Aspiration Pneumonia: Streptococcus pneumoniae, bacteroides sp., oral anaerobes, klebsiella, Enterobacter.

AIDS & PNEUMOCYSTIS CARINII PNEUMONIA

History: Progressive exertional dyspnea. Fever, chills, insidious onset of symptoms; CD4 lymphocyte count and percentage; duration of HIV positivity; prior episodes of PCP.

Dry nonproductive cough (or productive of white, frothy sputum), night sweats. Prophylactic trimethoprim/sulfamethoxazole treatment; antiviral therapy. Baseline and admission arterial blood gas.

Associated Symptoms: Headache, stiff neck, lethargy, fatigue, weakness, malaise, weight loss, diarrhea. Oral lesions, dysphagia, odynophagia (painful swallowing), weakness, altered mental status, skin lesions, visual changes.

Past Infectious Disease History: History of syphilis, herpes simplex, toxoplasmosis, tuberculosis, hepatitis. Prior influenza, pneumococcal immunization. Etiology of HIV infection; sexual and substance use history (intravenous drugs, blood transfusion).

Medications: Antivirals, prescribed and alternative medications.

Physical Exam:

General: Cachexia, respiratory distress.

Vitals: T (fever), R (tachypnea), P (tachycardia), BP (hypotension).

HEENT: Herpetic lesions; oropharyngeal thrush, hairy leukoplakia; oral Kaposi's sarcoma (purple-brown macules); retinitis, hemorrhages, perivascular white spots, cotton wool spots (CMV retinitis); visual acuity & visual field deficits (toxoplasmosis.)

Neck rigidity, lymphadenopathy.

Chest: Dullness, rhonchi, decreased breath sounds at bases; crackles.

Heart: Murmurs (IV drug users).

Abdomen: Right upper quadrant tenderness, hepatosplenomegaly.

Pelvic/Rectal: Candidiasis, anal herpetic lesions, ulcers, condyloma.

Dermatologic Stigmata of AIDS: Rashes, Kaposi's sarcoma (multiple purple nodules or plaques), seborrheic dermatitis, zoster, herpes, molluscum contagiosum; oral thrush.

Lymph Node Examination: Enlarged nodes.

Neuro: Confusion, disorientation (AIDS dementia complex, meningitis, encephalitis), motor, sensory, cranial nerves, ataxia, visual acuity and visual field deficits (toxoplasmosis).

Labs: CXR: diffuse, bilateral, interstitial infiltrates.

ABG: hypoxia, increased Aa gradient; respiratory alkalosis. CBC Sputum gram stain, Pneumocystis stain; LDH, CD4 count, hepatitis surface antigen and antibody, VDRL, toxoplasmosis titer, electrolytes.

MENINGITIS

History: Duration and degree of fever; chills, rigors; headache, neck stiffness; cough, sputum; lethargy, malaise, anorexia, irritability, confusion, nausea, vomiting. Nursing home or hospital acquired; skin rashes, myalgias, dysuria, ill contacts, travel history.

History of pneumonia, bronchitis, otitis media, sinusitis, endocarditis, cellulitis.

Diabetes, alcoholism, sickle cell disease, splenectomy malignancy, immuno-suppression, AIDS; recent upper respiratory infections, antibiotic use. History of intravenous drug use, tuberculosis.

Physical Exam:

General: Level of consciousness; obtundation, labored respirations.

Vitals: T (fever), P (tachycardia), R (tachypnea), BP (hypotension).

HEENT: Pupil size and reactivity, extraocular movements, papilledema. Brudzinski's sign (neck flexion causes hip and knee flexion); Kernig's sign (flexing hip and extending knee elicits resistance).

Chest: Rhonchi, crackles.

Heart: Murmurs.

Skin: Capillary refill, rashes; nail bed splinter hemorrhages, Janeway's lesions (Endocarditis), petechia, purpura (meningococcemia).

Neuro: Altered mental status, cranial nerve palsies, motor weakness, sensory deficits, Babinski's sign, gag reflex.

CT SCAN: Rule out increased intracranial pressure.

Labs: CSF: (see chart below). CBC, electrolytes, BUN, creatinine.

Differential Diagnosis: Meningitis, encephalitis, brain abscess, parameningeal infection, viral infection, tuberculosis. Cervical muscle strain, cervical disc disease, osteomyelitis, subarachnoid hemorrhage.

Etiology of Bacterial Meningitis:

15 - 50 years: Streptococcus pneumoniae, N. meningitis, listeria.

>50 years or debilitated: Same as above plus - Hemophilus influenza, Pseudomonas, streptococci.

AIDS: Cryptococcus neoformans, toxoplasma gondii, herpes encephalitis, coccidioides.

CEREBRAL SPINAL FLUID ANALYSIS

DISEASE	COLOR	PROTEIN	CELLS	SUGAR
Normal CSF Fluid	Clear	<50 mg/100 ml	<5 lymphs/mm^3	>40 mg/100 ml, 1/2-2/3 blood sugar drawn at same time
Bacterial meningitis early viral or tuberculous meningitis	Yellow opalescent	Elevated 50-1500	25-10000 WBC with predominate polys	low
Tuberculous, fungal, partially treated bacterial, syphilitic meningitis, meningeal metastases	Clear opalescent	Elevated usually <500	10-500 WBC with predominant lymphs	20-40, low
Viral meningitis, partially treated bacterial meningitis, & encephalitis, toxoplasmosis, parameningeal infection	Clear opalescent	Slightly elevated or normal	10-500 WBC with predominant lymphs	normal, may be low

PYELONEPHRITIS & URINARY TRACT INFECTION

History: Acute dysuria, frequency (voiding repeatedly of small amounts), urgency; suprapubic discomfort or pain, hematuria, malodorous or cloudy urine, fever, chills, malaise (pyelonephritis); aching back pain, nausea, vomiting.

History of urinary infections, renal stones or colicky pain. Recent antibiotic use, prostate enlargement. Internal or external dysuria sensation. Tampon use, bubble baths, long intervals between bladder emptying; diaphragm use.

Risk factors: Diaphragm or spermicide use, sexual intercourse, elderly, acquired anatomic abnormality, calculi, prostatic obstruction, confinement in bed, urinary tract instrumentation. Urinary tract obstruction, catheterization, anticholinergic drugs (urinary retention).

Physical Exam:

General: Signs of dehydration.

Vitals: T (fever), R (tachypnea), P (tachycardia), BP (hypotension if pyelonephritis).

Abdomen: Suprapubic tenderness, costovertebral angle tenderness, masses.

Pelvic/Genitourinary: Urethral or vaginal discharge, urethrocele.

Rectal: Prostatic hypertrophy or tenderness (prostatitis).

Labs: UA with micro. Urine Gram stain, urine C&S. CBC with differential, SMA7.

Pathogens: E coli, Klebsiella, Proteus, Pseudomonas, Enterobacter, Staphylococcus saprophyticus, enterococcus, group B strep, chlamydia trachomatis.

Differential Diagnosis: Acute cystitis, pyelonephritis, vulvovaginitis with or without gonococcal or chlamydia urethritis, herpes, cervicitis, urethral irritants, allergic urethritis, urinary tract obstruction, acute renal infarction, papillary necrosis, renal calculus, appendicitis, cholecystitis, vaginitis, pelvic inflammatory disease.

ENDOCARDITIS

History: Fever, chills, night sweats, weakness, fatigue, malaise; pain in fingers or toes; pleuritic chest pain; skin lesions, weight loss; history of heart murmur, rheumatic heart disease, heart failure, prosthetic valve.

Intravenous drug use; recent intravenous catheter, dental procedures; infection or instrumentation of urinary or gastrointestinal tract; colonic disease, decubitus ulcers, wound infection. History of stroke.

Physical Exam:

Vitals: T (fever), P (tachycardia), BP (hypotension).

HEENT: Oral mucosal and conjunctival petechiae; Roth's spots (retinal hemorrhages with pale center; emboli).

Heart: New or worsening cardiac murmur.

Abdomen: Liver tenderness (abscess); splenomegaly, spinal tenderness (vertebral abscess).

Neuro: Focal neurological deficits (septic emboli).

Extremities: Splinter hemorrhages under nails; Osler's nodes (erythematous or purple tender nodules on pads of toes or fingers); Janeway lesions (erythematous nontender lesions on palms and soles, septic emboli), joint pain (septic arthritis).

Labs: WBC, ESR; UA: hematuria; blood cultures, urine culture.

Echocardiogram: vegetation, valvular insufficiency.

CXR: cardiomegaly, valvular calcifications, prosthetic valve, infiltrate, effusion.

Pathogens:

Native Valve: Streptococcus viridans, streptococcus bovis, enterococci, staphylococcus aureus, streptococcus pneumonia, pseudomonas, group D streptococcus.

Prosthetic Valve: Staphylococcus aureus, Enterobacter sp., staphylococcus epidermidis, diphtheroids, candida, aspergillus.

GASTROENTEROLOGY

ACUTE ABDOMEN & ABDOMINAL PAIN

History: Duration of pain and pattern of progression; location at onset and at present; diffuse or localized; character at onset and at present (burning, gnawing, crampy, sharp, dull); constant or intermittent ("colicky"); radiation (right shoulder, left shoulder, mid-back, or groin); sudden or gradual onset. Effect of eating, vomiting, defecation, flatus, urination, inspiration, movement, position. Timing and characteristics of last bowel movement. Similar episodes in past. Relation to last menstrual period, pregnancy.

Associated Symptoms: Fever, chills, nausea, vomiting (bilious, feculent, undigested food, blood, coffee grounds); vomiting before or after onset of pain; chest pain, constipation, change in bowel habits or stool caliber, obstipation (inability to pass gas); diarrhea, dysuria, hematuria, hematochezia (rectal bleeding), melena (black stools); anorexia, weight loss, dysphagia, odynophagia (painful swallowing); early satiety, jaundice, trauma.

History of abdominal surgery (appendectomy, cholecystectomy, aortic graft), hernias, gallstones; coronary disease, kidney stones; alcoholism, ascites, dyspepsia.

Past treatment or testing: Endoscopies, x-rays, upper GI series, recent instrumentation.

Aggravating or Relieving Factors: Fatty food intolerance, medications, aspirin, NSAID's. Use of opiate narcotics, anticholinergics, laxatives, antacids.

Physical Exam:

General: Degree of distress; severity of pain; nutritional status. "Jack-knife posture".

Vitals: T (fever), P (tachycardia), BP (orthostatic hypotension), R (tachypnea).

HEENT: Pale conjunctiva, scleral icterus, atherosclerotic retinopathy, "silver wire" arteries (ischemic colitis); flat neck veins (hypovolemia). Lymphadenopathy, Virchow node (supraclavicular mass).

ABDOMEN:

Inspection: Scars, stria, evidence of trauma, ecchymosis, visible peristalsis (small bowel obstruction), distension. Scaphoid, flat, distended; exact point of maximal pain.

Auscultation: Absent bowel sounds (paralytic ileus or late obstruction), high-pitched rushes (obstruction); bruits (ischemic colitis).

Palpation: Begin palpation in quadrant diagonally opposite to point of maximal pain with patient's legs flexed and relaxed. Bimanual palpation of flank (renal disease or retrocecal appendix).

Rebound tenderness; hepatomegaly, splenomegaly, masses; hernias (incisional, inguinal, femoral). Pulsating masses; costovertebral angle tenderness. Bulging flanks, shifting dullness, fluid wave (ascites). Digital examination of stomas.

Specific Signs on Palpation: Murphy's sign (inspiratory arrest with right upper quadrant palpation, cholecystitis). Charcot's sign (right upper quadrant pain, jaundice, fever; gallstones). Courvoisier's sign (palpable, nontender gallbladder with jaundice, pancreatic malignancy).

McBurney's point tenderness (located two thirds of the way between umbilicus & anterior superior iliac spine, appendicitis). Iliopsoas sign (elevation of legs against examiner's hand causes pain, retrocecal appendicitis). Obturator sign (flexion of right thigh & external rotation of thigh causes pain in pelvic appendicitis).

Rovsing's sign (manual pressure and release at left lower quadrant colon causes referred pain at McBurney's point, appendicitis). Cullen's sign (bluish periumbilical discoloration, peritoneal hemorrhage). Grey Turner's sign (flank ecchymoses, retroperitoneal hemorrhage).

Percussion: Loss of liver dullness (perforated viscus, free air in peritoneum); liver and spleen span by percussion.

Rectal: Masses, tenderness, feces; gross or occult blood. Bimanual with on hand palpating lower abdomen for tenderness or mass.

Genital/Pelvic Examination: Adnexal tenderness, cervical discharge, uterine size, masses, cervical motion tenderness.

Extremities: Femoral pulses, popliteal pulses (absent pulses may indicate ischemic colitis) edema.

Skin: Jaundice, dependent purpura (mesenteric infarction), petechia (gonococcemia).

Stigmata of Liver Disease: Spider angiomata, periumbilical collateral veins (Caput medusae), gynecomastia, ascites, hepatosplenomegaly, testicular atrophy.

Labs: CBC, electrolytes, liver function tests, amylase, lipase, UA, pregnancy test. ECG.

Chest x-ray: free air under diaphragm, infiltration, effusion-left side pancreatitis.

X-rays of abdomen (acute abdomen series): flank stripe, subdiaphragmatic free air, distended loops of bowel, sentinel loop, "Double wall sign", air fluid levels, thumb printing, mass effect, calcifications, fecaliths, portal vein gas, pneumatobilia, aortic aneurysm.

Differential Diagnosis:

Generalized Pain: Intestinal infarction, generalized peritonitis, obstruction, diabetic ketoacidosis, sickle crisis, acute porphyria, penetrating posterior duodenal ulcer, psychogenic.

Right Upper Quadrant: Biliary colic, cholecystitis, cholangitis, hepatitis, gastritis, pancreatitis, hepatic metastases, gonococcal perihepatitis (Fitz-Hugh-Curtis syndrome), retrocecal appendicitis, pneumonia, peptic ulcer, gastroesophageal reflux disease.

Epigastrium: Gastritis, peptic ulcer, esophagitis, gastroenteritis, pancreatitis, perforated viscus, intestinal obstruction, ileus, myocardial infarction, aortic aneurysm.

Left Upper Quadrant: Peptic ulcer, gastritis, esophagitis, gastroesophageal reflux, pancreatitis, pericarditis, myocardial ischemia, pneumonia, splenic rupture/infarction, pulmonary embolus.

Left Lower Quadrant: Diverticulitis, intestinal obstruction, colitis, strangulated hernia, inflammatory bowel disease, gastroenteritis, pyelonephritis, nephrolithiasis, mesenteric lymphadenitis, mesenteric thrombosis, aortic aneurysm/rupture, volvulus, intussusception, sickle crisis, salpingitis, ovarian cyst, ectopic, testicular torsion, psychogenic.

Right Lower Quadrant: Appendicitis, diverticulitis (redundant sigmoid) salpingitis, endometritis, perforated Meckel's diverticulum, intussusception, ruptured ectopic pregnancy, hemorrhage or rupture of ovarian cyst, renal calculus, perforated cecal diverticulum, regional enteritis.

Hypogastric/Pelvic: Cystitis, salpingitis, ectopic, diverticulitis, endometriosis, appendicitis, ovarian cyst torsion; distended bladder, hernia, nephrolithiasis, pregnancy, prostatitis, carcinoma.

NAUSEA & VOMITING

History: Character of emesis (color, food, bilious, feculent, hematemesis, coffee ground material, projectile); vertigo, tinnitus (labyrinthitis); abdominal pain, effect of vomiting on pain, early satiety, fever, melena.

Clay colored stools, dark urine, jaundice (biliary obstruction); myalgias, recent change in medications. Ingestion of spoiled, contaminated food; regurgitation of undigested food, dysphagia, odynophagia.

Possibility of pregnancy (last menstrual period); exposure to Ill contacts, common food sources. Diabetes, cardiac disease, ulcer, liver disease, CNS disease, migraine headache.

Drugs Causing Nausea: Colchicine, digoxin, aminophylline, chemotherapy, alcohol, anticholinergics, morphine, Demerol, ergotamines, oral contraceptives, estrogen, antiarrhythmics, heavy metal poisoning, erythromycin, antibiotics.

Past Testing: X-rays of abdomen, upper GI series, endoscopy.

Physical Exam:

Vitals: BP (orthostatic hypotension), P (tachycardia), R, T (fever).

Skin: Temperature, pallor, jaundice, spider angiomas.

HEENT: Nystagmus, papilledema; ketone odor on breath (apple odor, diabetic ketoacidosis), uremic breath (fishy odor); jugular venous distention.

Abdomen: Scars, bowel sounds, bruits, tenderness, rebound, rigidity, distention, splenomegaly, hepatomegaly, ascites.

Extremities: Edema.

Rectal: Masses, occult blood.

Labs: CBC, electrolytes, UA, amylase, lipase, LFT's, acute abdomen x-ray series; pregnancy test.

Differential Diagnosis: Bacterial, vial, parasitic infections of GI tract, gastroenteritis, systemic infections, medications (contraceptives, antiarrhythmics, chemotherapy, antibiotics), pregnancy, appendicitis, cholecystitis, hepatitis, obstruction, peptic ulcer , gastroesophageal reflux, gastroparesis, ileus, pancreatitis, myocardial ischemia, constipation/obstipation, tumors (esophageal, gastric) increased intracranial pressure, labyrinthitis, diabetic ketoacidosis, renal failure, toxins, bulimia, psychogenic.

ANOREXIA & WEIGHT LOSS

History: Time of onset, amount and rate of weight loss (sudden, gradual); change in appetite, nausea, vomiting, dysphagia, abdominal pain; pain associated with eating (intestinal angina); diarrhea, fever, chills, sweats; dental problems; availability of food.

Polyuria, polydipsia, polyphagia; stress, anxiety; skin or hair changes, insomnia; 24-hour diet recall; dyspepsia, jaundice, dysuria; cough, change in bowel habits; chronic medical illness.

Dietary restrictions (low salt, low fat), misconceptions about nutrition; diminished taste. Malignancy, exposure to tuberculosis, AIDS risks factors; anorexia nervosa, psychiatric disease, suicidal ideation, renal disease; history of alcoholism, drug abuse (cocaine, amphetamines).

Vegetative signs of depression: Weight change, change in appetite, loss of interest in usual activities, sleep abnormalities, decreased libido.

Physical Exam:

General: Signs of malnutrition, muscle wasting.

Vitals: P (bradycardia), BP, R, T (hypothermia).

Skin: Pallor, jaundice, hair changes; skin laxity, cheilosis, dermatitis, glossitis (Pellagra).

HEENT: Poor dentition, oropharyngeal lesions, thyromegaly, glossitis, supraclavicular, temporal wasting, adenopathy (Virchow's node).

Chest: Crackles, rhonchi, barrel shaped chest.

Heart: Murmurs, S_3, displaced PMI.

Abdomen: Scars, decreased bowel sounds, tenderness, hepatomegaly splenomegaly. Periumbilical adenopathy (Sister Mary Joseph's sign), palpable mass.

Extremities: Edema, muscle wasting, lymphadenopathy.

Neuropathy: decreased sensation, poor proprioception.

Rectal: Occult blood, masses.

Labs: CBC, electrolytes, protein, albumin, pre-albumin, transferrin, thyroid studies, LFT's, toxicology screen.

Differential Diagnosis: Inadequate intake, peptic ulcer, depression, anorexia nervosa, dementia, hyper/hypothyroidism, cardiopulmonary disease, "cardiac cachexia or pulmonary cachexia," sedatives, psychotropics, digoxin, laxatives, thiazides, antibiotics, narcotics, hypogeusthesia (diminished taste), diminished olfaction, poor dental hygiene (loose dentures), cholelithiasis, gastric reflux, malignancy (gastric carcinoma), gastritis, hepatic or renal failure, febrile illnesses, alcohol or drug abuse. AIDS, mesenteric ischemia, pancreatic insufficiency.

DIARRHEA

History: Nature of onset, duration, frequency, timing of the diarrheal episodes. Volume of stool output (number of stools per hour or day), loose or watery stools; fever, malaise. Cramping, abdominal pain, tenesmus (urge to defecate), nausea, vomiting, ability to keep food or liquids down, bloating; lightheadedness, myalgias, arthralgias, headache, weight loss.

Stool Appearance: Quantity, buoyancy; presence of blood or mucus. blood, pus, oily, foul odor;

Recent ingestion of spoiled, raw, undercooked poultry (salmonella), milk, seafood (shrimp, shellfish); common sources (restaurant), travel history.

Effect of fasting on diarrhea (osmotic diarrhea-decreases with fasting, secretory diarrhea-unchanged with fasting), laxative abuse.

Ill contacts with diarrhea, diabetes, inflammatory bowel disease, alcoholism, hyperthyroidism; family history of coeliac disease. Sexual exposures, immunosuppressive agents, AIDS risk factors.

Stress related, daytime only diarrhea with mucous stools (irritable bowel syndrome).

Drugs and Substances That May Cause Diarrhea: Laxatives, magnesium-containing antacids, sulfa-containing compounds, antibiotics (erythromycin, clindamycin), alcohol., cholinergic agents (metoclopramide), colchicine, milk (lactase deficiency), candy, gum (sorbitol).

Physical Exam:

General: Signs of dehydration or malnutrition.

Vitals: BP (orthostatic hypotension), P (tachycardia), R, T (fever).

Skin: Skin turgor, capillary refill, pallor, jaundice; erythema nodosum (erythematous, tender nodules on anterior tibia), pyoderma gangrenosum (pustular ulcers with erythematous halo, inflammatory bowel disease). Kaposi sarcoma (AIDS).

HEENT: Oral ulcers (inflammatory bowel or coeliac disease), dry mucus membranes, cheilosis (cracked lips, riboflavin deficiency); glossitis (B12, folate deficiency). Oropharyngeal thrush (candida esophagitis - AIDS).

Abdomen: Hyperactive bowel sounds, tenderness, rebound, hepatomegaly guarding, rigidity. Distention, pulsatile masses.

Extremities: Back pain, arthritis, joint swelling (ulcerative colitis).

Rectal: Perianal or rectal ulcers, rectal tags, fistulas, hemorrhoids; sphincter tone, tenderness, masses, occult blood, pus. Sphincter reflex.

Neuro: Peripheral neuropathy (B6, B12 deficiency), decreased perianal sensation.

Labs: Electrolytes, Wright's stain for fecal leucocytes; cultures for enteric pathogens, ova and parasites x 3; clostridium difficile toxin. CBC with differential, calcium, albumen, flexible sigmoidoscopy.

Abdominal X-ray: Intestinal mucosa inflammatory changes, air fluid levels, dilation, pancreatic calcifications (pancreatitis).

Differential Diagnosis:

Osmotic Diarrhea: Laxatives, lactulose, lactase deficiency (gastroenteritis, sprue), other disaccharidase deficiencies, ingestion of mannitol, nasogastric tube feeding, sorbitol.

Secretory Diarrhea: Bacterial enterotoxins, viral infection; AIDS associated disorders (mycobacterial, HIV), Zollinger-Ellison syndrome, vasoactive intestinal peptide tumor, carcinoid tumors, medullary thyroid carcinoma, colonic villus adenoma, terminal ileal disease with bile salt malabsorption..

Exudative Diarrhea: Bacterial infection, Clostridium difficile, parasites, Crohn's disease, ulcerative colitis, diverticulitis, chemotherapy, intestinal ischemia, radiation injury, diverticulitis with or without abscess.

Diarrhea Secondary to Altered Intestinal Motility: Diabetic gastroparesis, adrenal insufficiency, hyperthyroidism, laxatives, antibiotics, cholinergics, irritable bowel syndrome, GI bleeding, post surgical disorders ("dumping syndrome"). Bacterial overgrowth (stasis related), overflow diarrhea because of constipation.

Diarrhea Secondary to Decreased Surface Absorption: Bowel resection, fistulas, celiac sprue, short bowel syndrome.

HEMATEMESIS & UPPER GASTROINTESTINAL BLEEDING

History: Duration and frequency of hematemesis (vomiting bright red blood or coffee ground material), volume of blood, recent hematocrit. Forceful retching prior to hematemesis (Mallory-Weiss tear). Abdominal pain, melena, hematochezia (bright red blood per rectum); history of ulcers, esophagitis, prior bleeding episodes. Ingestion of alcohol, aspirin, nonsteroidal anti-inflammatory agents, steroids, anticoagulants, PeptoBismol; nose bleeds, syncope, lightheadedness, nausea.

Weight loss, malaise, anorexia, early satiety, jaundice. History of liver/renal disease, varices, aortic or abdominal surgery.

Past testing: x-ray studies, endoscopy. Past treatment.

Nasogastric aspirate quantity and character; transfusions given in emergency room. Family history of liver, gastrointestinal disease or bleeding disorders.

Physical Exam:

General: Pallor, diaphoresis; cold, clammy extremities; agitation, confusion.

Vitals: Supine and upright pulse and blood pressure, (orthostatic hypotension); (resting tachycardia =10% blood volume loss; postural hypotension with increase pulse of 20 and decrease in systolic of 20=20-30% loss); oliguria <20 mL/h, T.

Skin: Delayed capillary refill, pallor; petechiae, ecchymosis. Stigmata of liver disease: (umbilical venous collaterals (caput medusae), jaundice, spider angiomas, parotid gland hypertrophy). Hemorrhagic telangiectasia (Osler-Weber-Rendu syndrome), abnormal pigmentation (Peutz-Jeghers syndrome); purple brown nodules (visceral Kaposi's sarcoma).

HEENT: Scleral pallor, oral telangiectasia, flat neck veins.

Chest: Gynecomastia (cirrhosis), breast masses (metastatic disease).

Heart: Systolic ejection murmur.

Abdomen: Scars, bowel sounds, tenderness, rebound, masses, splenomegaly, hepatomegaly, liver nodules. Ascites, dilated abdominal veins.

Extremities: Dupuytren's contracture (palmar contracture, cirrhosis), edema, bone pain (metastasis).

Neuro: Decreased mental status, confusion, poor memory, asterixis (flapping with wrists hyperextended, hepatic encephalopathy).

Genitourinary/Rectal: Gross or occult blood, masses; testicular atrophy.

Labs: CBC, electrolytes, BUN (↑ suggests upper GI bleed), glucose, PT/PTT, bleeding time; ECG. Endoscopy, nuclear scan, angiography.

Differential Diagnosis of Upper Bleeding: Gastric or duodenal ulcer, gastritis, esophagitis, esophageal varices, Mallory Weiss tear (gastroesophageal junction tear due to vomiting or retching), swallowed blood (nose bleed, oral lesion), duodenitis, malignancy (esophageal, gastric), vascular ectasias, carcinoid, coagulopathy, hypertrophic gastropathy (Menetrier's disease), aorto-enteric fistula.

MELENA & LOWER GASTROINTESTINAL BLEEDING

History: Duration, quantity, color of bleeding (gross blood, streaks on stool, toilet paper melena). Recent hematocrit. Change in bowel habits or stool caliber; abdominal pain, fever. Constipation, diarrhea; epistaxis (nose-bleeds); anorexia, weight loss, malaise; vomiting, nausea. Fecal mucus, pus, tenesmus (straining during defecation), lightheadedness; history of diverticulosis, hemorrhoids, colitis, peptic ulcer, heartburn, hematemesis, bleeding disease, colon polyps, aortic stenosis; coronary or renal disease, cirrhosis, alcoholism, anorectal pain, easy bruising.

Pepto Bismol or iron (black stools); red meat (false positive hemoccult). Antibiotics (pseudomembranous colitis), anticoagulants, aspirin, NSAIDS. Color of nasogastric aspirate.

Past Testing: Barium enema, colonoscopy, proctoscopy, upper GI series.

Physical Exam:

Vitals: BP, P (orthostatic hypotension, tachycardia), R, T; oliguria.

Skin: Cold, clammy skin; delayed capillary refill, pallor, jaundice. Stigmata of liver disease: Umbilical venous collaterals (Caput medusae), jaundice, spider angiomata, parotid gland hypertrophy, gynecomastia. Rashes, purpura; buccal mucosa discolorations or pigmentation (Henoch-Schönlein purpura or Peutz-Jeghers polyposis syndrome).

HEENT: Atherosclerotic retinal disease (ischemic colitis), narrowing, "silver wire" arteries.

Heart: Systolic ejection murmurs (aortic stenosis); atrial fibrillation (mesenteric emboli).

Abdomen: Scars, bowel sounds, bruits, masses, distention, rebound, tenderness, hernias, hepatomegaly, splenomegaly. Ascites, pulsatile masses (aortic aneurysm).

Genitourinary: Testicular atrophy.

Extremities: Cold, pale extremities; bone pain (metastasis).

Neuro: Decreased mental status; confusion, asterixis (flapping hand tremor, hepatic encephalopathy).

Rectal: Gross or occult blood, masses, hemorrhoids; fissure or tears, polyps, ulcers.

Labs: CBC (anemia), liver function tests. Upright abdomen x-ray (thumbprinting, air fluid levels, volvulus).

Differential Diagnosis of Lower Gastrointestinal Bleeding: Hemorrhoids,

fissures, diverticulosis, rectal trauma, proctitis, upper GI bleeding, inflammatory bowel disease, infectious or ischemic colitis, bleeding polyps, carcinoma,
vascular ectasias (angiodysplasias), intussusception, ulcerations,
coagulopathies, Meckel's diverticulitis, epistaxis small intestine tumor,
endometriosis, AV malformation.

CHOLECYSTITIS

History: Duration of biliary colic (constant right upper quadrant pain, occurring
30-90 minutes after meals, lasting several hours). May radiate to right
epigastrium, scapula or back; nausea, vomiting, anorexia, low grade fever;
fatty food intolerance, dark urine, clay colored stools; bloating, jaundice, early
satiety, increased belching, flatulence, obesity. Previous epigastric pain,
gallstones, alcohol. Fever, right upper quadrant pain, jaundice. History of
fasting, rapid weight loss high calorie diets, hyperalimentation, estrogen,
diabetes, sickle cell anemia, hereditary spherocytosis.

Risk Factors: "fair, fat, female, fertile, > forty." Hyperlipidemia. Previous
abdominal surgery.

Prior Testing: Ultrasounds, HIDA scans, endoscopies.

Pigment Stones: Asians with biliary parasites, hemolytic states (sickle cell
anemia, hereditary spherocytosis); cirrhosis, biliary stasis.

Cholesterol Stones: Hereditary, pregnancy, exogenous steroids use, diabetes
with gall bladder dysfunction; Crohn's disease, terminal ileal resection; rapid
weight loss, hyperalimentation.

Physical Exam:

General: Obese, restless patient unable to find comfortable position.

Vitals: P (mild tachycardia), T (low-grade fever), R (shallow respirations), BP.

Skin: Jaundice

HEENT: Scleral icterus, sublingual jaundice.

Abdomen: Epigastric or right upper quadrant tenderness, Murphy's sign
(increased tenderness and inspiratory arrest during deep palpation of RUQ);
firm tender, sausage-like mass in RUQ (enlarged gallbladder); guarding,
rigidity, rebound; Charcot's sign (intermittent right upper quadrant abdominal
pain, jaundice, fever).

Labs: Ultrasound, HIDA (radionuclide) scan, WBC, ↑ bilirubin, ↑ alkaline
phosphatase, AST (SGOT),amylase.

Plain Abdominal X-ray: ↑ gallbladder shadow, calcifications in gallbladder; air in gallbladder wall (emphysematous cholecystitis); biliary tree air (cholecystenteric fistula), small bowel obstruction (gallstone ileus).

Differential Diagnosis: Calculus cholecystitis, acalculous cholecystitis, biliary colic, cholangitis, peptic ulcer, pancreatitis, appendicitis, gastroesophageal reflux disease, hepatitis, abscess, nephrolithiasis, pyelonephritis, hepatic metastases, gonococcal perihepatitis (Fitz-Hugh-Curtis syndrome), pleurisy, pneumonia, angina, pericarditis, herpes zoster.

JAUNDICE & HEPATITIS

History: Dull right upper quadrant pain, or acute "colicky" right upper quadrant pain, anorexia, jaundice, nausea, vomiting, fever, shaking chills; diarrhea, dark urine, increased abdominal girth (ascites), pruritus, arthralgias, urticarial rash; somnolence, lethargy (hepatic encephalopathy). Weight loss, melena, hematochezia, hematemesis. IV drug abuse, alcoholism, exposure to hepatitis or jaundiced persons, blood transfusion, oral-fecal exposure, day care centers, residential institutions; prior hepatitis immunization.

Hepatotoxin Exposure: Acetaminophen, isoniazid, nitrofurantoin, methotrexate, sulfonamides, amiodarone, NSAIDS, phenytoin, methyldopa, phenothiazines, oral contraceptives.

Heart failure, recent sepsis or surgery. Family history of jaundice/liver disease.

Prior Testing: Hepatitis serologies, liver function tests, liver biopsy.

Physical Exam:

Vitals: P, BP, R, T (fever).

Skin: Needle tracks, sclerotic veins (from intravenous injections), urticaria, bronze discoloration (hemochromatosis).

Stigmata of liver disease: Jaundice, umbilical venous collaterals (Caput medusae), spider angiomas, palmar erythema.

HEENT: Scleral icterus, sublingual jaundice, lymphadenopathy, Kayser-Fleischer rings (bronze corneal pigmentation, Wilson's disease).

Chest: Gynecomastia, Murphy's sign (cessation of inspiration while examiner presses on right upper quadrant).

Abdomen: Scars, bowel sounds, right upper quadrant tenderness; liver span, hepatomegaly; liver margin texture (blunt, irregular, firm), spleen size, splenomegaly, ascites. Courvoisier's sign (palpable nontender gallbladder with jaundice - pancreatic or biliary malignancy).

Genitourinary: Testicular atrophy.

Extremities: Joint tenderness, arthritis, palmar erythema, Dupuytren's contracture (fibrotic palmar ridge to ring finger).

Neuro: Decreased mental status; disorientation, confusion, asterixis (flapping when wrists are hyperextended, encephalopathy).

Rectal: Occult blood; hemorrhoids.

Labs: CBC with differential, LFT's, amylase/lipase, hepatitis serologies (hepatitis B surface antibody, hepatitis B surface antigen, hepatitis A IgM, hepatitis C antibody), antimitochrondrial antibody (primary biliary cirrhosis), ANA, ceruloplasmin, urine copper (Wilson's disease), alpha 1 antitrypsin deficiency, drug screen, HIV, serum iron, TIBC, ferritin (hemochromatosis), pregnancy test (cholestasis of pregnancy, acute fatty liver), right upper quadrant ultrasound, ERCP, liver biopsy.

Differential Diagnosis of Jaundice:

Extrahepatic: Biliary tract disease (gallstone stricture, cancer), infections (parasites, AIDS, CMV/microsporidia); pancreatic disease (acute pancreatitis, chronic pancreatitis with stricture, pancreatic cancer, pseudocyst), porta hepatis lymphadenopathy.

Intrahepatic: Viral hepatitis, medication-related, pregnancy (acute fatty liver), alcoholic injury (hepatitis, cirrhosis), primary biliary cirrhosis, autoimmune hepatitis, Wilson's disease, right heart failure, total parenteral nutrition related; hereditary deficiency (increased direct hyperbilirubinemia - Dubin Johnson syndrome, Rotor's syndrome; indirect - Gilbert's, Crigler-Niger), sclerosing cholangitis (AID's, inflammatory bowel disease); infiltrative disease (Hodgkin disease, sarcoidosis, amyloidosis, tumor).

CIRRHOSIS

History: Jaundice, anorexia, nausea, fever; abdominal distension or pain, increased abdominal girth, weight gain; vomiting, diarrhea, malaise, fatigue, amenorrhea. Somnolence, confusion (encephalopathy); alcohol use. Viral hepatitis, hepatotoxin exposure, blood transfusion, IV drug use.

Precipitating Factors of Encephalopathy: Gastrointestinal bleeding, high protein intake, constipation, azotemia, hypokalemic alkalosis, CNS depressants.

Physical Exam:

General: Fetor hepaticas (odor of breath caused by mercaptans); muscle wasting.

Vitals: P, BP, T, R.

Skin: Jaundice, spider angiomas (stellate, erythematous arterioles), palmar erythema; bronze skin discoloration (hemochromatosis); purpura; loss of body hair.

HEENT: Kayser-Fleischer rings (bronze corneal pigmentation, Wilson's disease), jugular venous distention (fluid overload). Parotid enlargement, sclera icterus, gingival hemorrhage (thrombocytopenia).

Chest: Bibasilar crackles, gynecomastia.

Abdomen: Bulging flanks, tenderness, rebound (peritonitis); fluid wave, shifting dullness, "puddle sign" (examiner flicks over lower abdomen while auscultating for dullness). Courvoisier's sign (palpable nontender gallbladder with jaundice; pancreatic or Biliary malignancy); atrophic liver; liver margin texture (blunt, irregular, firm). Splenomegaly. Umbilical or groin hernias.

Genitourinary: Edema of scrotum or penis, testicular atrophy.

Extremities: Lower extremity edema.

Neuro: Confusion, asterixis (jerking movement of hand with wrist hyperextended), hepatic encephalopathy.

Rectal: Occult blood, hemorrhoids.

Stigmata of Liver Disease: Spider angiomas (stellate red arterioles), jaundice, bronze discoloration (hemochromatosis), dilated periumbilical collateral veins (Caput medusae), ecchymoses, umbilical eversion, venous hum and thrill at umbilicus or xiphoid (Cruveilhier-Baumgarten syndrome); palmar erythema, Dupuytren's contracture (fibrotic palmar ridge to ring finger). Lacrimal and parotid gland enlargement, Terry's nails (white proximal nail beds, cirrhosis), testicular atrophy, gynecomastia, hepatomegaly, splenomegaly, ascites, GI bleeding, encephalopathy, thin wasted extremities, bipedal edema.

Labs: CBC, electrolytes, LFT's, albumin, total protein, HIV, PT/PTT, liver function tests; UA. Hepatitis serologies, bilirubin, antimitochondrial, antibody (primary, biliary cirrhosis), ANA, anti-smooth muscle antibody, ceruloplasmin, urine, copper (Wilson's disease), alpha 1 antitrypsin, serum iron, TIBC, ferritin (hemochromatosis).

Abdominal x-ray: Hepatic angle sign (loss of lower margin of right, lateral, liver angle), separation or centralization, of bowel loops, generalized abdominal haziness. Ultrasound, paracentesis.

Differential Diagnosis:

Alcoholic liver disease, viral hepatitis (B, C, D), hemochromatosis, primary biliary cirrhosis, autoimmune hepatitis, inborn error metabolism (Crigler Najjar syndrome; Wilson's disease, alpha 1 antitrypsin deficiency), schistosomiasis, malnutrition, bypass surgery, chronic heart failure, venous outflow obstruction (Budd-Chiari, portal vein thrombus).

EVALUATION OF ASCITES FLUID:

Etiology	Appearance	Protein	Serum/fluid Albumen Gradient	RBC	WBC	Other
Cirrhosis	Straw/bile	<3 g/dL	>1.1	low	<250 cells/mm3	
Spontaneous Bacterial Peritonitis	Clear/cloudy	<3	>1.1	low	>250 polys	Bacteria on gram stain & culture
Secondary Bacterial Peritonitis	Purulent	>3	<1.1	low	>10000	Bacteria on gram stain & culture multiple organisms, bilirubin > 6.0
Neoplasm	Straw/bloody	>3	varies	high	>1000 lymphs	Malignant triglycerides; cells on cytology
Tuberculosis	Clear/bloody	>3	<1.1	low-high	>1000 lymphs	Acid fast bacilli
Heart failure	Straw	>3	>1.1	low	<1000	
Pancreatitis	Turbid/bloody	>3	<1.1	varies	varies	Elevated amylase, lipase
Myxedema	Clear/cloudy	>3	>1.1	low	<1000 WBC	

PANCREATITIS

History: Severe to mild, steady, boring, or penetrating, mid-epigastric pain; radiation to back; sudden onset; exacerbated by supine position, relieved by sitting with knees drawn up; nausea, vomiting, chills; fever, rigors, jaundice; anorexia, dyspnea; elevated amylase.

Precipitating Factors: Alcohol, gallstones, trauma, postoperative, retrograde cholangiopancreatography, trauma, hypertriglyceridemia, hypercalcemia, renal failure, viral (Coxsackie virus, mumps), or mycoplasma infection. Lupus, vasculitis, penetration of peptic ulcer, scorpion stings. Tumor, pancreatic division, sphincter of Oddi dysfunction.

Medications Associated with Pancreatitis: Sulfonamides, thiazides, chlorpropamide dideoxyinosine (DDI), furosemide, tetracycline, estrogens, azathioprine, valproate, pentamidine.

Physical Exam:

General: Signs of volume depletion, tachypnea.

Vitals: Low grade fever, tachycardia, hypotension.

Chest: Crackles, left lower lobe dullness (pleural effusion).

HEENT: Scleral icterus, Chvostek's sign (taping cheek results in facial spasm, hypocalcemia).

Skin: Jaundice, subcutaneous fat necrosis (erythematous skin nodules on legs and ankles, 1-10 mm in diameter). Palpable purpura (polyarteritis nodosum).

Abdomen: Epigastric or periumbilical tenderness; rigidity, rebound, guarding, hypoactive or silent bowel sounds; upper abdominal mass, distention; Cullen's sign (periumbilical bluish discoloration from hemoperitoneum), Grey-Turner's sign (blue or greenish flank discoloration, retroperitoneal hemorrhage).

Extremities: Peripheral edema, anasarca.

Labs: Amylase, lipase, calcium, WBC, triglycerides, glucose, AST, LDL, UA.

Abdomen X-Rays: Ileus, sentinel loop (spasm of transverse colon), pancreatic calcifications, obscure psoas margins, displaced or atonic stomach. Colon cutoff sign (spasm of splenic flexure with no distal colonic gas), diffuse ground-glass appearance of ascites.

Chest x-ray: Left plural effusion.

Ultrasound: Gallstones, pancreatic edema or enlargement.

CT scan: With oral contrast. Pancreatic phlegmon, pseudocyst, abscess.

Ranson's Criteria of Pancreatitis Severity.

Early criteria: Age >55; WBC >16,000; glucose >200; LDH >350 IU/L; AST >250.

During initial 48 hours: Hematocrit decrease >10%; BUN increase >5; arterial pO2 <60 mmHg, (on room air); base deficit >4 mEq/L; calcium <8; estimated fluid sequestration >6 L.

Differential Diagnosis of Midepigastric Pain: Pancreatitis, peptic ulcer, cholecystitis, hepatitis, bowel obstruction, strangulation of hernia, mesenteric ischemia, renal colic, aortic rupture/dissection, pneumonia, myocardial ischemia.

Causes of Pancreatitis: Alcoholic pancreatitis, gallstone pancreatitis, penetrating peptic ulcer, trauma, medications, hyperlipidemia, hypercalcemia (hyperparathyroidism), infections (viral, ascaris), congenital disorders (pancreatic divisum, familial pancreatitis), malignancy (pancreatic), toxins (methyl alcohol, scorpion bites), sphincter of Oddi dysfunction, endoscopic retrograde pancreatitis, vasculitis.

GASTRITIS & PEPTIC ULCER DISEASE

History: Recurring, dull, gnawing, burning, epigastric pain; 1-3 hours after meals; relieved by food or worsen by food; worse when supine or reclining; relieved by antacids; awakens patient at night or in early morning. May radiate to back; nausea, vomiting, weight loss; early satiety; hematemesis, coffee ground emesis; melena. Smoking, alcohol. Salicylates, nonsteroidal anti-inflammatory drugs, corticosteroids. Pre-existing cirrhosis, COPD, renal failure, stress; abdominal surgery.

History of previous examinations: Endoscopy upper GI series, surgery; history of previous ulcer disease; history of endocrine disorder - Men I syndrome (parathyroid, pituitary, pancreas, gastrinoma).

Physical Exam:

General: Mild distress.

Vitals: P, BP (orthostatic hypotension), R, T.

Skin: Pallor.

Abdomen: Mild to moderate epigastric tenderness; rebound, rigidity, guarding; scars, bowel sounds.

Rectal: Occult blood.

Labs: CBC, electrolytes, BUN, amylase. Abdominal x-rays, endoscopy.

Differential Diagnosis: Pancreatitis, gastritis, duodenitis, gastroenteritis, peptic ulcer, perforating ulcer, Crohn's disease with ulcer, intestinal obstruction, mesenteric adenitis, mesenteric thrombosis, aneurysm, gastric dysmotility, gastroesophageal reflux disease, non-ulcer dyspepsia.

MESENTERIC ISCHEMIA & INFARCTION

History: Severe, poorly localized, mid-abdominal pain; postprandial, relieved by nitroglycerine; accompanied by or followed within 24 hours by bloody diarrhea; food aversion; weight loss during preceding months, nausea, vomiting. Peripheral vascular disease, claudication, chest pain, coronary artery disease, atrial fibrillation, hypercholesterolemia; diabetes, autoimmune disease (SLE), nonocclusive hypotension, CHF.

Physical Exam:

General: Lethargy, mild to moderate distress.

Vitals: P, BP (orthostatic hypotension), P (tachycardia), R, T.

HEENT: Atherosclerotic retinopathy, "silver wire" arteries; carotid bruits (ischemic colitis).

Skin: Cold clammy skin, pallor.

Abdomen: Initially hyperactive, then followed by absent bowel sounds; distention, peritonital signs (rebound, tenderness, rigidity, guarding), pulsatile masses (aortic aneurysm), abdominal bruit.

Extremities: Weak peripheral pulses, femoral bruits; asymmetric pulses (atherosclerotic disease).

Rectal: Occult or gross blood.

Labs: CBC, electrolytes, leukocytosis. Hemoconcentration, prerenal azotemia, serum lactic acid (metabolic acidosis).

Chest x-ray: Free air under diaphragm (perforated viscus). Abdominal x-ray: "thumb-printing" (edema and gas of intestinal wall), portal vein gas. Bowel wall gas (colonic ischemia, nonocclusive); angiogram with surgical standby.

INTESTINAL OBSTRUCTION

History: Vomiting, obstipation, distention, crampy abdominal pain. Initially crampy or colicky pain with exacerbations at intervals of 5-10 minutes. Pain later becomes diffuse with fever. Hernias, previous abdominal surgery, use of opiates, anticholinergics, antipsychotics, tricyclics, gallstones; colon cancer; history of constipation, previous episodes of rectal bleeding, vomiting. Character of emesis (feculent, bloody). Pain localizes to periumbilical region in small bowel obstruction and localizes to lower abdomen in large bowel obstruction.

Physical Exam:
General: Severe distress.

Vitals: BP (hypotension), P (tachycardia), R, T (fever).

Skin: Cold clammy skin, pallor.

Abdomen: Hernias (incisional, inguinal, femoral, umbilical), scars.

Bowel Sounds: High pitch rushes or absent bowel sounds (late). Tenderness, rebound, rigidity, masses, distention. Hepatomegaly, bruits. Succussion splash (gastric outlet obstruction).

Rectal: Gross blood, masses.

Labs: CBC, electrolytes; metabolic alkalosis due to vomiting; or metabolic lactic acidosis. Amylase, pH, ABG.

Abdominal x-rays: dilated loops of small or large bowel, air-fluid levels, sentinel loop.

Differential Diagnosis:

Small Bowel Obstruction: Adhesions (previous surgery), hernias, strictures from inflammatory processes; superior mesenteric artery syndrome, gallstone ileus. Ischemia, primary small bowel tumors (adenocarcinoma, carcinoid, lymphoma, metastatic tumors (breast, melanoma, ovarian, colon).

Large Bowel Obstruction: Colon cancer, volvulus, diverticulitis, adynamic ileus, mesenteric ischemia, Ogilvie's syndrome (chronic pseudo-obstruction); narcotic ileus. Inflammatory bowel disease with stricture.

Differential Diagnosis: Myocardial infarction, gallstones, hiatal hernia, peptic ulcer, gastroenteritis, peritonitis, sickle crisis, cancer, pancreatitis, renal colic.

ALCOHOL WITHDRAWAL

History: Usual alcohol intake (number of drinks per day), time of last alcohol intake; tremors, anxiety, nausea, vomiting; chills, diaphoresis, agitation, fever, abdominal pain, headache; hematemesis, melena; seizures, past withdrawal reactions; history of delirium tremens, blackouts, hallucinations, binge drinking; chest pain.

Past Medical History: Gastritis, ulcers, GI bleeding; hepatitis, cirrhosis, ascites, tuberculosis, AIDS, pancreatitis, drug abuse. Age of onset of heavy drinking, family history of alcoholism.

Physical Exam:

General: Poor nutritional status, slurred speech, disorientation, hyperactivity, diaphoresis.

Vitals: BP (hypertension), P (tachycardia), R, T (hyper/hypothermia).

HEENT: Signs of head trauma, ecchymoses. Conjunctival injection, icterus, nystagmus, extraocular movements, pupil reactivity, anisocoria (unequal pupil size). Battle's sign (ecchymosis of mastoid process, basilar skull fracture).

Chest: Rhonchi, crackles (aspiration), gynecomastia (cirrhosis).

Heart: Rate and rhythm, murmurs.

Abdomen: Liver tenderness, hepatomegaly, liver span, splenomegaly, ascites.

Genitourinary: Testicular atrophy, hernias.

Rectal: Occult blood.

Skin: Jaundice, spider angiomas (stellate arterioles with branching capillaries), palmar erythema, Dupuytren's contracture, muscle atrophy (stigmata of liver disease).

Neuro: Cranial nerves 2-12, asymmetric reflexes or hyperreflexia, ataxia. Asterixis, sensory deficits, decreased vibration sense (peripheral neuropathy).

Wernicke's Encephalopathy: Ophthalmoplegia; ataxia, global confusion (secondary to thiamine deficiency).

Korsakoff's Syndrome: Retrograde/antegrade amnesia; confabulation.

Labs: Electrolytes, magnesium, glucose, blood alcohol, CBC, bilirubin, liver tests folate; chest X-ray; ECG, UA, CT scan, lumbar puncture.

Differential Diagnosis of Altered Mental Status: Acute alcohol intoxication, hypoglycemia, meningitis, pneumonia, drug overdose, toxic ingestion, head trauma, hypothermia, alcoholic ketoacidosis, acute schizophrenia, drug-induced psychosis, anticholinergic poisoning, sedative-hypnotic withdrawal, intracranial hemorrhage, hepatic or Wernicke's encephalopathy.

GYNECOLOGY

AMENORRHEA

History: Primary amenorrhea (absence of menses by age 16) or secondary amenorrhea (cessation of menses for 6 months in a female with previously normal menstruation. Determine the menstrual pattern, timing of pubertal milestones, sexual activity (possibility of pregnancy).

Life style changes; dietary and exercise habits; medications or drugs; environmental and psychologic stress.

History of dilation and curettage, postpartum infection or hemorrhage (Sheehan's syndrome), obesity, weight gain or loss; head injury; headaches, visual disturbances, thyroid symptoms; symptoms of pregnancy, phenothiazines, Aldomet, antidepressants, opiates, hormones

Hot flushes, night sweats, and dyspareunia (decreased estrogen effects). Galactorrhea.

Family history of amenorrhea or genetic anomalies.

Physical Exam: Secondary sexual characteristics, body dimensions and habitus, inguinal or labial masses, papilledema, optic atrophy, signs of hyper/hypothyroidism. Galactorrhea, obesity; thyroid enlargement; breast atrophy; breast development, vaginal obstruction, uterine enlargement, ovarian cysts or tumors.

Evidence of increased androgen (acne, hirsutism, temporal balding, deepening of the voice, increased muscle mass, and decreased breast size).

Labs: Pregnancy test, prolactin, TSH, free T_4. Progesterone-estrogen challenge testing.

Differential Diagnosis: Hypogonadotropic or hypothalamic disfunction (psychogenic, anorexia nervosa, stress), endocrine disease, (estrogen or androgen secreting tumors; polycystic ovarian syndrome), outflow tract abnormalities. Intrauterine synechiae (Asherman's syndrome), primary ovarian failure (Gonadal dysgenesis), acquired ovarian failure (autoimmune, irradiation, infection), secondary ovarian failure (pituitary prolactinoma).

ABNORMAL UTERINE BLEEDING

History: Last menstrual period, menarche; regularity, duration/frequency of menses; number of pads per day; passing of clots; postcoital or intermenstrual bleeding, vasomotor flushing; changes in hair or skin texture or distribution; pain, fever, chills, lightheadedness; possibility of pregnancy, birth control method.

Molimina symptoms (mid-cycle ovulatory pain, premenstrual breast tenderness, water retention, dysmenorrhea). Obstetrical history.

Systemic diseases, particularly thyroid, renal, or hepatic diseases, coagulopathies. Medications associated with hyperprolactinemia (antidepressants, psychotropics, methyldopa). Dental bleeding, stress, exercise, weight changes.

Family history of coagulopathies, endocrine disorders.

Physical Exam: Assess hemodynamic stability, rate of bleeding. Orthostatic vitals; cervical lesions; skin and hair changes, thyroid enlargement, galactorrhea. Obesity, hirsutism, petechiae. Clitoromegaly, cervical motion tenderness, uterine size, cervical lesions, adnexal tenderness.

Cervical lesions should be evaluated with a Pap smear and biopsy.

Labs: CBC, platelets; serum pregnancy test, Pap smear; GC and chlamydia cultures, endometrial sampling. LFT's, thyroid panel; prolactin (if ovulatory dysfunction possible), PT/PTT, type and screen.

Differential Diagnosis: Anovulatory uterine bleeding (hypothalamic-pituitary dysfunction, polycystic ovarian syndrome), pregnancy-related (threaten abortion, postpartum, ectopic, gestational trophoblastic disease), malignancies (vulvar, vaginal, cervix, uterus, ovarian), ovarian hormone-producing tumors, endometrial hyperplasia, leiomyomata, endometrial or endocervical polyps, infectious disease (vaginitis, cervicitis, pelvic inflammatory disease), trauma; intrauterine device, medications (estrogen, progesterone, phenothiazines, tricyclic antidepressants, oral contraceptives, propanolol, digoxin, cyproheptadine, metoclopramide, cimetidine), systemic diseases (coagulation disorders, Cushing's syndrome, thyroid disease, liver disease).

PELVIC PAIN AND ECTOPIC PREGNANCY

History: Positive pregnancy test; missed menstrual period, pelvic or abdominal pain (bilateral or unilateral), symptoms of pregnancy; abnormal uterine bleeding or amenorrhea. Menstrual and obstetrical history.

Characteristics of pelvic pain; onset, duration; palliative/aggravating factors; shoulder pain. Rupture of ectopic pregnancy usually occurs between 6-12 weeks after last menstrual period.

Associated Symptoms: Urinary or gastrointestinal symptoms, fever, vaginal discharge.

Past Medical History: Surgical history, gynecologic history, pelvic inflammatory disease, ectopic pregnancy, sexually transmitted diseases.

Method of Contraception: Oral contraceptives or barrier method, intrauterine device (IUD).

Risk Factors for Ectopic Pregnancy: Prior pelvic infection, endometriosis, prior ectopic pregnancy, pelvic tumor, intrauterine device, pelvic/tubal surgery, infertility, diethylstilbestrol exposure in utero.

Risk Factors for Acute Pelvic Inflammatory Disease: Age between 15-25 years, use of an intrauterine device, male sexual partner with symptoms of urethritis, prior history of acute PID.

Physical Exam:

General: Moderate to severe distress.

Vitals: BP (orthostatic hypotension), P (tachycardia), R, T (low fever).

Skin: Cold clammy skin, pallor.

Abdomen: Hypoactive bowel sounds, Cullen's sign (periumbilical darkening, intra abdominal bleeding), local then generalized tenderness, bowel sounds, tenderness, rebound.

Pelvic: Cervical motion tenderness; Chadwick's sign (cervix and vaginal cyanosis, pregnancy); Hegar's sign (softening of uterine isthmus, pregnancy); enlarged uterus; tender pelvic/adnexal mass or cul-de-sac fullness.

Labs: Quantitative beta-HCG, transvaginal ultrasound. Type and hold, Rh, CBC, UA with micro.

Differential Diagnosis: Intrauterine pregnancy, salpingitis, endometriosis, ectopic pregnancy, appendicitis, threatened abortion, dysmenorrhea, dysfunctional uterine bleeding, ovarian cyst (corpus luteum), ovarian torsion, urinary tract infection, renal stone, diverticulitis, mesenteric lymphadenitis.

NEUROLOGY

HEADACHE

History: Duration, quality (dull, band-like, sharp, throbbing), location (bilateral or unilateral), time course of typical headache episode; onset (gradual or sudden); exacerbating or relieving factors; time of day, periodicity, effect of supine posture.

Age at onset of headaches; change in severity, frequency; awakening from sleep; family history of migraine; excess analgesic or codeine use. "The worst headache ever" (subarachnoid hemorrhage).

Aura or Prodrome: Scotomata; scintillating, zig-zag lines, blurred vision; nausea, vomiting; sensory disturbance.

Associated Symptoms: Numbness, weakness, diplopia, photophobia, fever; neck stiffness (meningitis), syncope; eye pain or redness (glaucoma); ataxia, dysarthria, transient blindness; facial, jaw pain or claudication (temporal arteritis).

Aggravating or Relieving Factors: Relief by analgesics or sleep. Exacerbation by foods (chocolate, alcohol, wine, cheese, tyramine), emotional upset, menses; hypertension, food allergies, trauma, drugs, cocaine; lack of or excess sleep; exacerbation by fatigue, exertion, sex (coital cephalgia), monosodium glutamate, nitrates. Occupational toxins (carbon monoxide).

Drugs: Nitrates, calcium blockers, phenothiazines, sedatives, theophylline, sympathomimetics, estrogen, MAO inhibitors, cotrimoxazole, corticosteroids, excessive ergotamine, cold remedies, eye drops, diet pills, cocaine.

Pain free periods, lacrimation, flushing, periodicity (cluster headaches).

Neck or back pain. Sinusitis

Symptoms of Depression: Sleep disturbance, decreased energy, loss of interest in usual pleasurable activities, poor concentration, sadness. Weight loss, decreased appetite, suicidal ideation.

Physical Exam:

Vitals: BP (hypertension), P, T (fever), R.

HEENT: Cranial or temporal tenderness or thickening of temporal artery (temporal arteritis), asymmetric pupils or reactivity; papilledema, loss of venous pulsations; extraocular movements, visual field deficits. Conjunctival injection, lacrimation, rhinorrhea (cluster headache).

Jaw or temporomandibular joint tenderness (TMJ syndrome); temporal/ocular bruits (arteriovenous malformation); sinus tenderness.

Dental infection, tooth tenderness to percussion; tympanic membrane inflammation; mastoid ecchymosis "battle's sign"; paraspinal muscle tension.

Neck: Neck rigidity.

Skin: Facial "peau d'orange" skin (cluster headache); petechiae, stria; cafe au lait spots (neurofibromatosis); adenoma sebaceum (facial angiofibromas); hypopigmented ash leaf spots (tuberous sclerosis), herpetic lesions (zoster).

Neuro: Cranial nerve palsies (intracranial tumor); auditory acuity, focal weakness, tendon reflexes, ataxia.

Labs: Electrolytes, ESR, MRI scan, lumbar puncture. CBC with differential, PT/PTT.

Indications for MRI scan: Focal neurologic signs, papilledema, decreased visual acuity, increased frequency or severity of headache, excruciating or paroxysmal headache, awakening from sleep, persistent vomiting; recurrent morning headache, head trauma with focal neurologic signs or lethargy.

Differential Diagnosis: Migraine, tension headache; systemic infection, subarachnoid hemorrhage, drug related, sinusitis, arteriovenous malformation, malignant hypertension, temporal arteritis, meningitis (viral, bacterial, fungal), encephalitis, post concussion syndrome, intracranial tumor, venous sinus thrombosis, benign intracranial hypertension (pseudotumor cerebri), subdural hematoma, trigeminal neuralgia, post-herpetic neuralgia, facial pain, glaucoma, pheochromocytoma, brain abscess, analgesic overuse, psychogenic, food allergy, hypoxia, anemia, hyper/hypothyroidism..

Migraine: Childhood to early adult onset; usually a family history; aura of scotomas or scintillations, unilateral pulsating or throbbing pain; nausea, vomiting. Lasts 2-6 hours; relief with sleep. Triggered by wine, cheese, chocolate, contraceptives, exercise, travel, menstruation, stress, lack of sleep.

Tension Headache: Bilateral, generalized, bitemporal or suboccipital. Band-like pressure; may throb, and occurs late in day; related to stress. Onset in adolescence or young adult; nonfamilial. Lasts hours and usually relieved by simple analgesics.

Cluster Headache: Recurrent, unilateral, retroorbital searing pain. Lacrimation, nasal and conjunctival congestion. Young males; lasts 20-60 min. Occurs in clusters at same time of night or several times each day over several weeks; followed by pain-free periods of months or years.

DIZZINESS & VERTIGO

<u>History:</u> Sensation of spinning or movement of surroundings; faintness and lightheadedness, nausea, vomiting, tinnitus. Rate of onset and intensity of vertigo. Aggravation by change in position, turning head, changing from supine to standing, coughing, urination. Effect of motion on symptoms.

Hyperventilation, postural unsteadiness. Poor vision, recent change in eyeglasses. Headache, vomiting, diarrhea, melena, diaphoresis, hearing loss, head trauma.

<u>**Associated Symptoms:**</u> Recent upper respiratory infection; dysarthria, diplopia, paresthesias, syncope; hypertension, diabetes, history of stroke, transient ischemic attack, anemia, cardiovascular disease, ear infections, hypertension.

Drugs causing vertigo: Antihypertensives, aspirin, alcohol, sedatives, diuretics, phenytoin, ototoxic drugs (gentamicin, neomycin).

<u>**Physical Exam:**</u>

<u>General:</u> Affect of Valsalva maneuver; hyperventilation may provoke symptoms.

<u>Vitals:</u> P, BP (supine and upright, postural hypotension), R, T.

<u>**HEENT:**</u> Nystagmus, visual acuity; visual field deficits; papilledema; facial weakness or sensory loss. Tympanic membrane inflammation (otitis media), cerumen. Effect of head turning, or of placing the patient recumbent with head extended over edge of bed; Rinne's test (air/bone conduction); Weber test (lateralization of sound).

<u>Heart:</u> Rhythm, murmurs.

<u>Neuro:</u> Cranial nerves 2-12; confusion, sensory deficits, ataxia, weakness, cranial nerve palsies, Babinski's sign. Romberg test, coordination (finger to

nose test), tandem gait.

Rectal: Occult blood.

Labs: CBC, electrolytes. MRI scan.

Differential Diagnosis:

Drugs Associated with Vertigo: Aminoglycosides, loop diuretics, aspirin, caffeine, alcohol, phenytoin, psychotropics (lithium, haloperidol), benzodiazepines. Volatile hydrocarbons, anesthetics, solvents.

Peripheral Causes of Vertigo: Acute Labyrinthitis/Neuronitis, benign positional vertigo, Meniere's disease (vertigo, tinnitus, deafness), otitis media, acoustic neuroma, cerebellopontine angle tumor, cholesteatoma (chronic middle ear effusion), impacted cerumen.

Central Causes of Vertigo: Vertebrobasilar insufficiency, brain stem or cerebellar infarctions, tumors. Brain stem encephalitis, meningitis; skull fracture; brain stem/cerebellar contusion. Parkinsonism, multiple sclerosis and other demyelinating diseases.

Other Disorders Associated with Vertigo: Motion sickness, presyncope, syndrome of multiple sensory deficits (peripheral neuropathies, visual impairment, orthopedic problems); altered visual input (new glasses); orthostatic hypotension.

DELIRIUM, COMA AND CONFUSION

History: Level of consciousness; obtundation (awake but not alert), stupor (unconscious but awakable with vigorous stimulation), coma (cannot be awakened). Confusion, hallucination, formification (sensation that insects are crawling under skin); delirium, tremor, poor concentration, agitations.

Activity and symptoms prior to onset. Use of insulin, oral hypoglycemics, narcotics, alcohol, drugs, antipsychotics, anticholinergics, cimetidine, anticoagulants; history of trauma, suicide attempts or depression; prior epilepsy (post-ictal state).

Fever, headache. History of dementia, stroke, transient ischemic attacks, hypertension; renal, liver, cardiac disease.

Physical Exam:

General: Signs of dehydration.

Vitals: BP (hypertensive encephalopathy), P, T (fever), R.

HEENT: Skull palpation for tenderness, lacerations. Pupil size and reactivity. Extraocular movements, corneal reflexes. Papilledema, venous pulsations, hemorrhages, flame lesions; ocular/temporal bruits, facial asymmetry, ptosis, weakness. Battle's sign (ecchymosis over mastoid process), Raccoon sign (periorbital ecchymosis, skull fracture), hemotympanum (basal skull fracture). Tongue or cheek lacerations (post-ictal state). Signs of B12 deficiency (pallor, atrophic tongue).

Neck: Neck rigidity, carotid bruits; lymphadenopathy.

Chest: Breathing pattern (Cheyne-Stokes hyperventilation); crackles, wheezes.

Heart: Rhythm, murmurs.

Abdomen: Hepatomegaly, splenomegaly, masses, ascites, tenderness, distention, dilated superficial veins (liver failure).

Extremities: Track marks (drug overdose).

Skin: Cyanosis, jaundice, spider angiomata, palmar erythema (hepatic encephalopathy); capillary refill, petechia, splinter hemorrhages. Localized fat atrophy (diabetic).

Neuro: Concentration (subtraction of serial 7's, indicates delirium) Strength, cranial nerves 2-12, mini-mental status exam; orientation to person, place, time, recent events; coordination, Babinski's sign, primitive reflexes (snout, suck, glabella, palmomental grasp). Tremor (Parkinson's disease, delirium tremens), incoherent speech, lethargy, somnolence.

GLASGOW COMA SCALE

Best Verbal Response: None - 1; Incomprehensible sounds or cries - 2; Appropriate words or vocal sounds - 3; Confused speech or words - 4; Oriented speech - 5

Best Eye Opening Response: No eye opening - 1; Eyes open to pain - 2; Eyes open to speech - 3; Eyes open spontaneously - 4

Best Motor Response: None - 1; Abnormal extension to pain - 2; Abnormal flexion to pain - 3; Withdraws to pain - 4; Localizes to pain - 5; Obeys commands - 6

Total Possible Score: 3-15

Special Neurologic Signs:

Decortication: Painful stimuli causes flexion of arms, wrist and fingers with leg extension; indicates damage to contralateral hemisphere above midbrain.

Decerebration: Painful Stimuli Causes extension of legs and arms; wrists and fingers flex with midbrain and pons functioning.

Oculocephalic Reflex: (Doll's eyes maneuver) Observation of eye movements in response to lateral rotation of head; no eye movements or loose movements occurs in bihemispheric (diencephalon) lesion.

Oculovestibular Reflex: (Cold caloric maneuver) Raise head 60 degrees and irrigate ear with cold water; causes tonic deviation of eyes to irrigated ear if intact brain stem; if conscious, causes nystagmus, vertigo, emesis.

Labs: Glucose, electrolytes, calcium, BUN, creatinine, ABG. CT/MRI, ammonia, alcohol, liver function tests, urine toxicology screen, B-12, folate levels. LP.

Differential Diagnosis of Delirium: Electrolyte imbalance, hyperglycemia/hypoglycemia (insulin overdose), alcohol/drug withdraw or intoxication, hypoxia, meningitis/encephalitis, systemic infection, stroke, intracranial hemorrhage, postictal state; exacerbation of dementia; narcotic or anticholinergic overdose; steroid withdrawal, hypotension, hepatic encephalopathy; psychotic states, dehydration, hypertensive encephalopathy; head trauma, subdural hematoma, uremia, vitamin deficiencies, hypothyroidism, factitious coma, ketoacidosis.

WEAKNESS & ISCHEMIC STROKE

History: Rate and pattern of onset of weakness (gradual, sudden); time course to maximum deficit, and time of onset; anatomic location of deficit; activity prior to onset (Valsalva, exertion); improvement or progression of symptoms; prior headache; nausea, vomiting, loss of consciousness; brisk neck movement; visual aura, scotoma, vertigo; seizure, trauma.

Confusion, dysarthria, incontinence, dysphagia, palpitations; prior transient ischemic attacks (neurologic deficit lasting longer than 24 hours) or strokes (permanent neurologic deficit); transient monocular blindness (Amaurosis fugax).

Past Medical History: Hypertension, diabetes, coronary disease, endocarditis, hyperlipidemia, IV drug abuse, cocaine use, heart failure, valvular disease, arrhythmias (atrial fibrillation), claudication, migraine, anticoagulants, oral contraceptives, alcohol, antihypertensives, cigarette smoking.

Past testing: CT scans, carotid Doppler studies, echocardiograms.

Family history: Stroke, hyperlipidemia, cardiac disease.

Physical Exam:

General: Level of consciousness, lethargy.

Vitals: BP (both arms), P (bradycardia), T, R. Cushing's response (bradycardia, hypertension, abnormal respirations).

HEENT: Signs of head trauma, pupil size and reactivity, extraocular movements. Fundi: hypertensive retinopathy; "bright plaques" (bright yellow retinal flecks, cholesterol emboli); Roth spots (flame shaped lesions, endocarditis), subhyaloid retinal hemorrhages (blood pocket indicating subarachnoid hemorrhage); papilledema, absent venous pulsations; facial asymmetry and weakness.

Neck: Neck rigidity, carotid bruits; asymmetrical carotid pulse amplitude (carotid artery disease); vertebrobasilar bruits (base of neck).

Chest: Breathing pattern, Cheyne Stokes respiration (periodic breathing with periods of apnea, elevated intracranial pressure).

Heart: Irregular, irregular rhythm (atrial fibrillation), S3 (heart failure), murmurs (mitral stenosis, cardiogenic emboli).

Abdomen: Aortic pulsations, renal bruits (atherosclerotic disease).

Extremities: Unequal peripheral pulses.

Skin: Petechia, splinter hemorrhages.

Neuro: Motor deficits, gag reflex, cranial nerves 2-12, gaze, ptosis, Babinski's sign (stroke sole of foot, and toes dorsiflex if pyramidal tract lesion); coordination. Clonus, primitive reflexes (snout, glabella, palmomental, grasp). Mini-mental status exam, memory concentration.

Signs of Increased Intracranial Pressure: Lethargy, headache, vomiting, meningismus, cranial nerve palsy, visual changes, gait disturbances, papilledema, absent venous pulsations, focal neurologic deficits, abnormal vital signs, seizures, hyperreflexia, head tilt.

Signs of Cerebral Herniation: Obtundation, dilation of ipsilateral pupil, decerebrate posturing (extension of elbows, wrists and legs; ascending weakness. Cushing's response - bradycardia, hypertension, abnormal respirations.

Labs: CT scan: bleeding, infarction, mass effect, midline shift. ECG, CBC.

Differential Diagnosis of Stroke Syndromes: Infection (abscess, meningitis, encephalitis), subdural hematoma, brain tumor, metabolic imbalance (hypoglycemia, hypocalcemia), demyelinating disease, vasculitis, postictal paralysis (Todd's paralysis), delirium; conversion reaction; atypical migraine, basilar artery stenosis, carotid steal syndrome, transient ischemic attack.

SEIZURE

History: Time of onset of seizure, duration, type (tonic-clonic), description of seizure. Past seizures; compliance with anticonvulsants (recent blood level). Aura (irritability, behavioral change, lethargy), pallor, incontinence of urine or feces; salivation, vomiting; aspiration, post-ictal weakness or paralysis.

Prodrome (visual changes, paresthesias), history of transient ischemic attacks, stroke, migraine headaches, fever, chills. Complex motor activities (lip smacking, leg movement), diabetes (hypoglycemia); family history of epilepsy.

Factors that May Precipitate Seizure: Fatigue, sleep deprivation, infection, hyperventilation, head trauma, alcohol withdrawal, cocaine. Meningitis, febrile seizure; drug or alcohol withdrawal, uremia; hypocalcemia, hypoglycemia, theophylline toxicity, stroke.

Substances Associated with Seizures: Phenothiazines, lithium, lidocaine, anticholinergics, alcohol, antidepressants, amphetamines, insulin, oral hypoglycemics (hypoglycemia), theophylline.

Past testing: EEG's, CT scans.

Physical Exam:

General: Post-ictal lethargy.

Vitals: BP (hypertension), P, R, T (hyperpyrexia).

HEENT: Evidence of head trauma; pupil reactivity and equality, extraocular movements; visual fields; papilledema, absent venous pulsations; gum hyperplasia (phenytoin); tongue or buccal lacerations; ocular, temporal bruits, carotid bruits, neck rigidity.

Chest: Rhonchi, wheeze (aspiration).

Heart: Rhythm, murmurs.

Extremities: Cyanosis, bone pain, fractures.

Genitourinary/Rectal: Incontinence of urine/feces.

Skin: Café-au-lait spots, neurofibromas (Von Recklinghausen's disease), splinter hemorrhages (endocarditis). Unilateral port-wine facial nevus (Sturge-Weber syndrome); facial angiofibromas (adenoma sebaceum), hypopigmented ash leaf spots, (tuberous sclerosis). Spider angiomas (hepatic encephalopathy), malar rash (lupus).

Neuro: Dysarthria; ability to follow commands; sensory deficits, visual fields, focal weakness (Todd's paralysis), coordination, cranial nerves, Babinski's sign (plantar responses).

Labs: Glucose, electrolytes, BUN, calcium, magnesium, liver function test, CBC, urine toxicology, blood alcohol, anticonvulsant levels, RPR/VDRL. EEG, MRI scan, lumbar puncture.

Differential Diagnosis: Epilepsy (complex partial seizure disorder, generalized tonic/clonic seizure disorder), noncompliance with anticonvulsants, hypoglycemia, hyponatremia, hypocalcemia, hypomagnesemia, hypertensive encephalopathy, alcohol/barbiturate withdrawal, meningitis, encephalitis, uremia, pyridoxine deficiency, trauma, brain tumor, congenital malformation, stroke, hepatic failure, uremia, vasculitis, pseudo-seizure.

NEPHROLOGY

OLIGURIA, ANURIA AND ACUTE RENAL FAILURE
ASSESSMENT OF VOLUME STATUS

History: Oliguria: <20 mL/h, 400-500 mL urine/day; anuria <100 mL urine/day; hemorrhage, heart failure, hypotension, sepsis, infection, vomiting, nasogastric suction; diarrhea, diuretics, sweating from fever; measure fluid input and output; history of Foley catheter obstruction, prostate enlargement, kidney stone, bladder disease, anticholinergics, opiates, recent use of bladder catheter.

Nephrotoxic drugs (aminoglycosides, neomycin, amphotericin, NSAID's), dysuria, urgency, flank pain. Abdominal pain; fever, chills, change in urine color, character, hematuria, passing of tissue fragments, foamy urine (proteinuria). Administration of renal by excreted medications.

Recent upper respiratory infection (post streptococcal glomerulonephritis), toxemia, recent chemotherapy (tumor lysis syndrome).

Physical Exam:

Vitals: BP (orthostatic vitals), P (tachycardia); an increase in heart rate by >15 mmHg and a fall in systolic pressure >15 mmHg, indicates significant volume depletion; T, R (tachypnea).

Skin: Decreased skin turgor over sternal angle (hypovolemia); skin temperature and color; jaundice (hepatorenal syndrome).

HEENT;Oral mucous membrane moisture; flat neck veins (volume depletion); venous distention (heart failure).

Chest: Crackles (rales, heart failure); basilar dullness to percussion (pleural effusion).

Heart: S3 (volume overload); cardiac friction rub (pericarditis).

Abdomen: Hepatomegaly, abdominojugular reflex; distended bladder, costovertebral angle tenderness, nephromegaly (hydronephrosis from obstruction).

Pelvic: Pelvic masses, cystocele, urethrocele.

Rectal: Prostate hypertrophy, occult blood; absent sphincter reflex and decreased sensation (atonic bladder due to vertebral disk herniation).

Extremities: Peripheral edema (sacral or pedal edema/anasarca).

Labs: Serum sodium, potassium, BUN, creatinine, uric acid. Urine and serum osmolality, UA, urine creatinine. Ultrasound of bladder and kidneys.

$$\text{Fractional excretion of sodium (FE Na)} = \frac{U_{Na}(mMol/L)}{S_{Na}(mMol/L)} \times \frac{S_{Cr}(mMol/L)}{U_{Cr}(mMol/L)} \times 100$$

$$\text{Renal Failure Index} = \frac{U_{Na} \times 100}{U/P_{Cr}}$$

TABLE OF PRE-RENAL, RENAL, POST-RENAL FAILURE:

	Prerenal	ARF	Postrenal
BUN/Creatinine ratio	715:1	<15:1	varies
Urine sodium	<20 mMol/L	720	varies
Urine osmolality	>500 mOsm/kg	<350	varies
Renal failure Index	<1	>1	varies
FE NA	<1%	>1%	varies
Urine/plasma creatinine	>40	>20	varies
Urine analyses	normal	cellular casts	RBC's, WBC's, bacteria

Differential Diagnosis:

Prenatal Failure:

Decreased Extracellular Volume with Decreased Intravascular Volume: Gastrointestinal loss (vomiting, diarrhea, nasogastric suction), dehydration, burns, hemorrhage.

Decreased Intravascular Volume with Increased ECF Volume: Cirrhosis; nephrotic syndrome, heart failure, third spacing of fluid (pancreatitis).

Hemodynamically Medicated Acute Renal Failure: NSAID associated ACE inhibitor, hepatorenal syndrome.

Intrinsic Acute Renal Failure:

Glomerular Disease: Glomerulonephritis/glomerulosclerosis

Tubulointerstitial Disease: Hypersensitivity reactions, associated with systemic infections, toxic exposures (organic solvents).

Acute Tubular Necrosis: Hypotension, septicemia, drug toxicity: aminoglycosides, amphotericin, cisplatin, contrast agents, cyclosporin, myoglobinemia/hemoglobinemia, toxemia of pregnancy.

Vascular Disease: Renal artery stenosis, vasculitis, hypertension, atheroembolic disease.

Postrenal Failure:

Intratubular Obstruction: Uric acid nephropathy, methotrexate.

Ureteric Obstruction: Retroperitoneal tumor (pelvic, prostate), retroperitoneal fibrosis.

Intrinsic: Nephrolithiasis, necrotic papillae, blood clot.

Ureteral Obstruction: Benign prostatic hypertrophy, blood clot, bladder dysfunction.

CHRONIC RENAL FAILURE

History: Oliguria, current and baseline creatinine and BUN. Diabetes, hypertension; history of urinary infection, sepsis, hemorrhage, heart failure, dyspnea, liver disease, peripheral edema; dark colored urine, rashes or purpura; new medications (nonsteroidal anti-inflammatory drugs, aminoglycosides, contrast dyes). Hypovolemia secondary to diarrhea, vomiting, hemorrhage, over-diuresis, glomerulonephritis, vasculitis, interstitial nephritis.

Past ultrasounds, dysuria, frequency, flank pain, history of kidney stones, prostate disease, urethral obstruction. Anorexia, insomnia, malaise, weight loss, bleeding, paresthesias, anemia, fatigue.

History of pathologic fractures, chronic flank pain. Family history of polycystic kidney disease, hereditary glomerulonephritis.

Physical Exam:

General: Evaluate intravascular volume status.

Vitals: Postural blood pressure and pulse (tachycardia, hypertension), T (fever), R.

Skin: Skin turgor, sallow yellow complexion (urochromes), fine white powder (uremic frost), purpura, petechiae (coagulopathy). Jaundice, spider angiomas (hepatorenal syndrome).

HEENT: Neck vein distention (volume overload).

Chest: Crackles (rales).

Heart: S3 gallop (volume overload), cardiac friction rub, displacement of heart border, muffled heart sounds (effusion), arrhythmias (electrolyte imbalances).

Abdomen: Distended bladder, costovertebral, or suprapubic tenderness, pelvic masses, ascites.

Rectal: Occult blood, prostate enlargement.

Neuro: Asterixis, myoclonus, decreased sensation.

Labs: BUN, creatinine, potassium (hyperkalemia), albumin, lipids, calcium, phosphorus, proteinuria.

Differential Diagnosis of Chronic Renal Failure: Hypertensive nephrosclerosis, diabetic nephrosclerosis, glomerulonephritis, polycystic kidney disease, tubulointerstitial renal disease, reflux nephropathy, analgesic abuse, chronic obstructive uropathy, amyloidosis, Lupus.

HEMATURIA

History: Frequency, dysuria, pain, colic, fever, fatigue, anorexia; abdominal, flank, or perineal pain. Exercise, jogging, menstruation; bleeding between voidings.

Foley catheter, prior stones; tissue passage, joint pain.

Color, timing, pattern of hematuria: initial hematuria (anterior urethral lesion); terminal hematuria (bladder neck or prostate lesion); hematuria throughout voiding (bladder or upper urinary tract).

Recent sore throat, streptococcal skin infection, upper respiratory infection (glomerulonephritis). Prior kidney infections, joint pain; travel to areas endemic for Schistosoma hematobilia; occupation exposure to toxins.

Family History: Hematuria, renal disease, sickle cell, bleeding diathesis, deafness (Alport's syndrome), hypertension.

Medications & Foods Associated with Hematuria: Warfarin, aspirin, ibuprofen, naproxen, indomethacin, penicillin, cephalexin, cephalothin, thiazides, furosemide, phenobarbital, allopurinol, phenytoin, cyclophosphamide.

Medications and Other Causes of Red Urine: Pyridium, phenytoin, ibuprofen, chloroquine, cascara laxatives, levodopa, methyldopa, quinine, nitrofurantoin, rifampin, sulfamethoxazole, berries, flava beans, food coloring, rhubarb, hemoglobinuria, myoglobinuria, mushrooms, sulfonamides, carbon monoxide, beets.

Physical Exam:

Vitals: BP (hypertension).

Skin: Rashes.

HEENT: Pharyngitis, rhinorrhea; carotid bruits.

Heart: Heart murmur; irregular, irregular (atrial fibrillation, renal emboli).

Abdomen: Tenderness, masses, costovertebral angle tenderness (renal calculus or pyelonephritis), abdominal bruits, nephromegaly, suprapubic tenderness, urethral tenderness.

Genitourinary: Urethral lesions, discharge, condyloma, foreign body, cervical malignancy; prostate tenderness, nodules, or enlargement (prostatitis).

Extremities: Peripheral edema (nephrotic syndrome), arthritis, ecchymoses, petechiae, weak or unequal peripheral pulses (aortic dissection).

Labs: UA with microscopic exam of urinary sediment, CBC, KUB (stones), intravenous pyelogram, ultrasound. Streptozyme panel, ANA, PT/PTT.

Indications for Evaluation: (1) >3 RBC's per high-power field on 2 of 3 specimens; (2) >100 RBC's per HPF in 1 specimen; (3) gross hematuria
Abstain from exercise 48 hours prior to collection and do not collect during menses.

Differential Diagnosis: Renal calculi, urinary neoplasm, tuberculosis, trauma, glomerulonephritis, papillary necrosis, analgesic nephropathy, hemoglobinopathies, prostatitis, cystitis, pyelonephritis, menstrual contamination, urologic endometriosis, allergic tubulointerstitial nephritis secondary to drugs; vasculitis (Wegener's granulomatosis), polyarteritis nodosa, immune-complex disorders (lupus, Goodpasture's syndrome), coagulopathies, urethritis, polycystic kidney disease, sickle cell disease, hypertension.

NEPHROLITHIASIS

History: Severe, colicky, intermittent, migrating, lower abdominal pain; hematuria, fever, dysuria; prior history of renal stones. Pain not associated with position; flank pain; abdominal pain may radiate laterally around abdomen to groin, testicles or labia. Time of last void; history of low fluid intake, urinary tract infection.

Calcium administration, immobilization, furosemide, neurogenic bladder, instrumentation of urinary tract; chemotherapy; family history of kidney stones. Inflammatory bowel disease, ileal resection. Diet high in oxalate: spinach, rhubarb, nuts, tea, cocoa. Excess vitamin C, hydrochlorothiazide; unusual dietary habits.

Physical Exam: Costovertebral angle tenderness, suprapubic tenderness; enlarged kidney.

Labs: Serum calcium, phosphorus bicarbonate, creatinine, uric acid. Urine cystine, UA microscopic (hematuria), urine culture, intravenous pyelogram.

Differential Diagnosis: Nephrolithiasis, cystitis, diverticulitis, appendicitis, salpingitis, hernia, ovarian torsion (cyst or mass), distended bladder, prostatitis, endometriosis, ectopic pregnancy, colon obstruction, inflammatory bowel disease, carcinoma (colon, prostrate, cervix, bladder).

Differential Diagnosis of Nephrolithiasis: Hypercalcemia, hyperuricosuria, hyperoxaluria, cystinuria, distal renal tubular acidosis (type 1), infection related Proteus mirabilis with staghorn calculi.

HYPERKALEMIA

History: Serum potassium of >5.5 mMol/L (repeat test to assure accuracy); muscle weakness, syncope, lightheadedness, palpitations, oliguria; excess intake of oral or intravenous potassium, salt substitutes, potassium sparing diuretics, angiotensin converting enzyme inhibitors; nonsteroidal anti-inflammatory drugs, beta blockers, heparin, digitalis toxicity, administration of potassium salts of penicillin; muscle or soft tissue trauma, chemotherapy (tumor lysis syndrome), cyclosporine, succinylcholine.

History of renal disease, diabetes, adrenal insufficiency (Addison's syndrome). History of episodes of paralysis precipitated by exercise (familial hyperkalemic periodic paralysis).

Physical Exam:

Skin: Hyperpigmentation (Addison's disease), hematomas.

Abdomen: Tenderness, suprapubic tenderness.

Neuro: Muscle weakness, abnormal deep tendon reflexes, cranial nerves 2-12.

Labs: Potassium, platelets, bicarbonate, chloride, anion gap, LDH, bilirubin, urine K, pH. Serum aldosterone, plasma renin activity.

ECG: Tall peaked, precordial T waves; QT interval is normal or diminished; widened QRS complex, prolonged PR interval, P wave flattening, AV block, ventricular arrhythmias, sine wave, asystole.

Differential Diagnosis:

Inadequate Excretion: Renal failure, adrenal insufficiency (Addison's syndrome), potassium sparing diuretics (spironolactone), urinary tract obstruction, lupus, hypoaldosteronism, ACE inhibitors, NSAIDs, heparin.

Increased Potassium Production: Hemolysis, rhabdomyolysis, muscle crush injury, internal hemorrhage, drugs (succinylcholine, digoxin poisoning, beta blockers), acidosis, hyperkalemic periodic paralysis, hyperosmolality.

Excess Intake of Potassium: Oral or IV potassium supplements, salt substitutes.

Pseudo-hyperkalemia: Hemolysis after collection of blood, excessively small needle, shaking of sample, delayed transport of blood to lab, thrombocytosis ($>10^5$ platelets/mm^3), leukocytosis ($>50,000$/mm^3), prolonged tourniquet use while drawing blood.

HYPOKALEMIA

History: Potassium <3.5; mMol/L (verified by repeat testing); hyperglycemia; diuretics, diarrhea, vomiting, laxative abuse; poor intake of potassium containing foods; corticosteroids, nephrotoxins, bicarbonate, insulin, beta agonists. Conn's syndrome (hyperaldosteronism).

Associated Symptoms: Muscle weakness, cramping pain, nausea, vomiting, constipation, palpitations, paresthesias, paralysis, cardiac arrest, polyuria.

Precipitating Factors: Renal disease, stress (catecholamine release), cell proliferation (B12 treatment); biliary drainage, enteric fistula; Kayexalate ingestion, dialysis, excessive licorice ingestion (chewing tobacco).

Physical Exam:

Vitals: BP, P, T, R.

Heart: Rate and rhythm.

Abdomen: Hypoactive bowel sounds (ileus), tenderness.

Neuro: Weakness, hypoactive tendon reflexes.

Labs: Serum potassium, spot urine potassium (>20 indicates renal loss); glucose. Plasma renin activity. Urine specific gravity, osmolality, CBC, electrolytes, BUN, creatinine, magnesium.

ECG: Flattening and inversion of T-wave (II, V3), ST segment depression, U waves (II, V1, V2, V3); 1st or 2nd degree block, QT interval prolongation, premature atrial/ventricular contractions, supraventricular tachycardia, ventricular tachycardia/fibrillation.

Differential Diagnosis of Hypokalemia:

Cellular Redistribution of Potassium: Intracellular shift of potassium by insulin (exogenous or glucose load), beta2 agonist; stress induced catecholamine release, thyrotoxic periodic paralysis; alkalosis-induced shift (metabolic or respiratory); familial periodic paralysis, barium intoxication; cellular proliferation (vitamin B12 treatment); hypothermia; acute myeloid leukemia.

Nonrenal Potassium Loss:

Gastrointestinal: Diarrhea, laxative abuse, villous adenoma, biliary drainage, enteric fistula, potassium binding resin ingestion

Sweating; prolonged low potassium ingestion; hemodialysis and peritoneal dialysis

Renal Potassium Loss:

Hypertensive High Renin States: Malignant hypertension, renal artery stenosis, renin-producing tumor.

Hypertensive Low Renin, High Aldosterone States: Primary hyperaldosteronism (adenoma or hyperplasia).

Hypertensive Low Renin, Low Aldosterone States: Congenital adrenal hyperplasia, Cushing's syndrome or disease, exogenous mineralocorticoids (Florinef, licorice, chewing tobacco), Liddle's syndrome

Normotensive: Renal tubular acidosis (type I or II); metabolic alkalosis (U Cl < 10 mEq/day)--vomiting; metabolic alkalosis (U Cl > 10 mEq/day): Bartter's syndrome, diuretics, magnesium depletion, normotensive hyperaldosteronism

HYPONATREMIA

History: Serum sodium <135 mMol/L; decreased mental status, apathy confusion, agitation, irritability, lethargy, anorexia, nausea, vomiting, headache, muscle weakness/tremor, cramps, seizure; decreased output of dark urine (dehydration); polydipsia (water intoxication), or dehydration; diuretics, diarrhea, steroid withdrawal.

Renal, CNS or pulmonary disease (syndrome of inappropriate antidiuretic hormone); heart failure, cirrhosis; hypotonic IV fluids; oral hypoglycemics (chlorpropamide), psychotropic medications, antineoplastics, hyperalimentation, hypothyroidism. Low sodium diet, excessive fluid intake; hyperlipidemia.

Physical Exam:

Vitals: BP, P (orthostatic vitals), T, R.

Skin: Decreased turgor, delayed capillary refill; hyperpigmentation (Addison's disease), moon-face, truncal obesity (hypoadrenalism with steroid withdrawal).

HEENT: Poor ocular and oral moisture.

Chest: Cheyne-Stokes respirations, crackles.

Heart: Rhythm and rate. Premature ventricular contractions.

Abdomen: Ascites, tenderness, costovertebral angle tenderness.

Extremities: Edema.

Neuro: Confusion, irritability. Motor weakness, ataxia, positive Babinski's sign, muscle twitches; hypoactive deep tendon reflexes, cranial nerve palsies.

Labs: Electrolytes, BUN, creatinine, cholesterol, triglycerides, glucose, protein, osmolality, albumin; CXR, ECG.

Differential Diagnosis of Hyponatremia Based on Urine Osmolality:

   A **Low Urine Osmolality (50-180 mOsm/L):** Primary excessive water intake (psychogenic water drinking).

   B **High Urine Osmolality (urine osmolality >serum osmolality):**

      1. **High Urine Sodium (>40 mEq/L) and Volume Contracted:** Renal source of fluid loss (excessive diuretic use, salt-wasting nephropathy, Addison's disease, osmotic diuresis).

      2. **High Urine Sodium (>40 mEq/L) and Normal Volume:** Water retention caused by a drugs (chlorpropamide, carbamazepine, amitriptyline, cyclophosphamide), hypothyroidism, syndrome of inappropriate antidiuretic hormone secretion.

      3. **Low Urine Sodium (<20 mEq/L) and Volume Contraction:** Extrarenal source of fluid loss (gastrointestinal disease, burns).

      4. **Low Urine Sodium (<20 mEq/L) and Volume-expanded, Edematous:** Heart failure, cirrhosis with ascites, and nephrotic syndrome.

HYPERNATREMIA

History: Serum sodium >145 mEq/L. History of dehydration due to fever, vomiting, burns, heat exposure, diarrhea, hyperventilation, severely elevated glucose, salt ingestion, administration of hypertonic fluids (sodium bicarbonate, sodium chloride, high osmolar enteral feedings), sweating; impaired access to water, adipsia (lack of thirst); head injury.

Altered mental status, lethargy, agitation, polyuria, anorexia, muscle twitching, renal disease. Recent IV fluid intake. Drugs causing hypernatremia: Amphotericin, phenytoin, lithium, aminoglycosides.

Physical Exam:

General: Lethargy, obtundation, stupor.

Vitals: BP (orthostatic hypotension), P (tachycardia), T, R; decreased urine output.

Skin: Decreased skin turgor ("doughy" consistency), delayed capillary refill, hyperpigmentation (Addison's disease), moon-face, truncal obesity, stria (hypoadrenal crisis, steroid withdrawal).

HEENT: Dry mucous membranes; flat neck veins, reduced eye turgor.

Neuro: Decreased muscle tone, ataxia, tremor, hyperreflexia; extensor plantar reflexes (Babinski's sign), tonic spasms, spasticity.

Labs: Increased hematocrit; sodium, BUN, creatinine, urine and serum, osmolality. 24 hour urine sodium, creatinine.

Differential Diagnosis:

Hypernatremia with Hypovolemia Due to Extrarenal Loss of Water (urine sodium >20 mMol/L): Vomiting, diarrhea; sweating, pancreatitis, respiratory loss. Renal loss of water (urine sodium <10 mMol/L): diuretics, hyperglycemia, renal failure.

Euvolemic Hypernatremia Renal Water Losses: Diabetes insipidus (central or nephrogenic).

Hypernatremia with Hypervolemia (urine sodium >20 mMol/L): Hypertonic solutions of sodium chloride or bicarbonate, hyperaldosteronism, Cushing's syndrome, congenital adrenal hyperplasia, dialysis.

ENDOCRINOLOGY

DIABETIC KETOACIDOSIS

History: Level of initial glucose, ketones, anion gap. Polyuria, polyphagia, polydipsia, fatigue, nausea, vomiting, weight loss; noncompliance with insulin and diet; blurred vision, emotional or physical stress, infection, dehydration., abdominal pain

Cough, fever, chills, ear infection, dysuria, frequency; back, chest or abdominal pain; dyspnea, nausea, vomiting, pregnancy.

Factors that May Precipitate Diabetic Ketoacidosis: New onset of diabetes, noncompliance with insulin, acute illness (infection, pancreatitis, myocardial infarction), stress, trauma, stroke, pregnancy.

History of infections, renal disease, myocardial infarction, stroke, gastroparesis; prior ketoacidosis, foot ulcers, decreased sensation in extremities (diabetic neuropathy), retinopathy, hypertension.

Physical Exam:

General: Decreased level of consciousness. Kussmaul respirations (deep sighing breathing).

Vitals: BP (orthostatic hypotension), P, T (fever or hypothermia), R (tachypnea).

Skin: Decreased turgor, delayed capillary refill; hyperpigmented atrophic macules on legs (shin spots); intertriginous candidiasis, erythrasma, localized fat atrophy (insulin injections).

HEENT: Diabetic retinopathy (neovascularization, hemorrhages, exudates); acetone breath odor (musty, apple-like odor), decreased visual acuity, low oral moisture (dehydration) tympanic membrane inflammation (otitis media); flat neck veins, neck rigidity.

Chest: Rales, rhonchi.

Abdomen: Hypoactive bowel sounds (ileus); gastric dilation (gastroparesis); tenderness, costovertebral angle tenderness, suprapubic tenderness (urinary tract infection).

Extremities: Decreased pulses, foot ulcers (examine between toes), cellulitis.

Neuro: Delirium, confusion; peripheral neuropathy (proprioception in feet), hypotonia, hyporeflexia.

Labs: Glucose, sodium, potassium, bicarbonate, chloride, BUN, creatinine, anion gap; triglycerides, phosphate, CBC; serum ketones, UA (proteinuria, ketones).

CXR, ECG.

Differential Diagnosis:

Ketosis-Causing Conditions: Alcoholic ketoacidosis or starvation.

Acidosis-Causing Conditions:

Increased Anion Gap: DKA, lactic acidosis, uremia, and poisoning from salicylates or methanol.

Non-Anion Gap: Renal or gastrointestinal electrolyte losses due to diarrhea or renal tubular acidosis.

Hyperglycemia-Causing Conditions: Hyperosmolar nonketotic coma.

Diagnostic Criteria for DKA: Glucose ≥ 250, pH <7.3, bicarbonate <15, ketone positive >1:2 dilutions.

HYPOTHYROIDISM & MYXEDEMA COMA

History: Lethargy, cold intolerance, constipation; weight gain or inability to lose weight, muscle weakness; thyroid swelling or mass; decreased exercise tolerance, dyspnea on exertion; mental slowing, dry hair and skin, deepening of voice; carpal tunnel syndrome, amenorrhea.

Past history of hyperthyroidism, thyroid testing, thyroid surgery or radioactive iodine treatment, antithyroid medication; exposure to iodine, lithium, amiodarone. Somnolence, apathy. Emotional lability, depression. Myxedema madness: agitation, disorientation, delusions, hallucinations, paranoia, restlessness, lethargy.

Family history of thyroid disease

Factors Predisposing to Myxedema Coma: Cold exposure, infection, trauma, surgery, anesthesia, narcotics, phenothiazines, phenytoin, sedatives, propranolol, alcohol.

Physical Exam:

General: Hypoactivity, confusion, somnolence; coarse, deep voice; dull, expressionless face.

Vitals: Bradycardia, hypotension, hypothermia.

Skin: Cool, dry, pale, rough, doughy skin; thin, brittle nails (dry with longitudinal ridges); yellowish skin without scleral icterus (carotenemia). Hyperkeratosis of elbows and knees; decreased sweat production.

HEENT: Thin, dry, brittle hair, alopecia; macroglossia (enlarged tongue), puffy face and eyelids; loss of lateral third of eyebrows; thyroid enlargement, thyroid scar. Jugular venous distention (pericardial effusion).

Chest: Dullness to percussion (pleural effusion).

Heart: Muffled heart sounds (pericardial effusion); displacement of lateral heart border; decreased intensity of point of maximal impulse, cardiomegaly, bradycardia.

Abdomen: Hypoactive bowel sounds (ileus), ascites (myxedema ascites).

Extremities: Bulky muscles with diminished strength and power. Myxedema: transient local swelling after tapping a muscle.

Neuro: Hypoactive tendon reflexes with delayed return phase. Decreased mental status, stupor, ataxia; visual field deficits, peripheral neuropathy, paresthesias, weakness.

Labs: Thyroid stimulating hormone, CBC, electrolytes, cholesterol ($\uparrow$), triglycerides ($\uparrow$), creatinine phosphokinase, LDH. ECG: bradycardia, low voltage QRS complexes; flattened or inverted T waves, prolonged Q-T interval.

Differential Diagnosis of Hypothyroidism: Autoimmune thyroid disease (Hashimoto's thyroiditis, atrophic hypothyroidism), iatrogenic (surgery, radioactive iodine therapy, antithyroid medications), iodine excess or deficiency, amiodarone, lithium; hypothalamic or pituitary radiation, tumor or surgery.

HYPERTHYROIDISM & THYROTOXICOSIS

History: Tremor, nervousness, hyperkinesis (restlessness), fever, heat intolerance, irritability, palpitations, diaphoresis, insomnia; thyroid enlargement, masses, thyroid pain; oligomenorrhea, amenorrhea.

Weight loss with increased appetite; dyspnea and fatigue (especially after slight exertion); softening of skin; fine, silky hair texture; proximal muscle weakness (especially thighs when climbing stairs).

Palpitations, atrial fibrillation; diplopia, reduced visual acuity; eye discomfort or pain, lacrimation; recent upper respiratory infection, hyperdefecation. Previous thyroid function testing; family history of thyroid disease.

Factors Precipitating Thyroid Storm: Infection, surgery, diabetic ketoacidosis, pulmonary embolus, excess hormone medication, cerebral vascular accident, myocardial infarction, labor and delivery, iodine -131 or iodine therapy.

Physical Exam:

General: Restless, anxious, hyperactive patient; delirium.

Vitals: Widened pulse pressure, hyperpyrexia (>104°F), tachycardia, hypertension.

Skin: Moist, warm, velvety skin, diaphoresis; palmar erythema, fine silky hair. Plummer's nails (distal onycholysis, separation of fingernail from nail bed), acropachy (clubbing of fingers and toes). Loss of subcutaneous fat and muscle mass.

HEENT: Exophthalmos (forward displacement of the eyeballs, proptosis), proptosis, widened palpebral fissures; lid lag and retraction, infrequent blink. Ophthalmoplegia (restricted extraocular movements), chemosis (edema of conjunctiva), conjunctival injection, corneal ulcers; periorbital edema or ecchymoses; optic nerve atrophy, impaired visual acuity, difficulty with convergence; fine tongue tremor.

Neck: Painless, diffusely enlarged, soft, rubbery thyroid without masses; thyroid thrill and bruit.

Heart: Irregular, irregular rhythm (atrial fibrillation), systolic murmur (mitral or tricuspid regurgitation, flow murmur), displacement of apical impulse, cardiomegaly. Accentuated first heart sound.

Extremities: Fine tremor; non-pitting pre-tibial edema (Grave's disease).

Neuro: Proximal muscle weakness, hyperreflexia (rapid return phase of deep tendon reflexes), rapid speech.

Labs: Thyroid tests: T4, TSH, beta-HCG.

ECG: Sinus tachycardia, atrial fibrillation.

Differential Diagnosis: Grave's disease, toxic multinodular goiter, acute thyroiditis, thyrotoxicosis factitia (ingestion of thyroid hormone), trophoblastic tumor (molar pregnancy), TSH producing adenoma, chronic or postpartum thyroiditis, ectopic thyroid tissue (struma ovarii, functional follicular carcinoma), thyroid adenoma/carcinoma.

HEMATOLOGY & RHEUMATOLOGY

DEEP VEIN THROMBOSIS

History: Unilateral calf pain; sudden onset of swelling and redness; exacerbation of pain by walking and flexing of foot; dyspnea.

Risk Factors: Virchow's triad: Immobilization, trauma, malignancy, (pancreas, lung, genitourinary, stomach, breast); estrogens (oral contraceptives), heart failure; prolonged bedrest, recent stroke, recent travel, history of deep vein thrombosis, pulmonary embolism. Obesity, pregnancy, lupus. History of surgery, nephrotic syndrome, polycythemia Vera, inflammatory bowel disease, antithrombin III deficiency, protein C deficiency.

Past Medical History: Abdominal pain, peptic ulcer, melena, bleeding risk factors, recent surgery.

Physical Exam:

Vitals: BP, P, R (dyspnea if pulmonary embolus), T (low-grade fever).

Chest: Breast masses.

Abdomen: Distention, tenderness, masses.

Genitourinary/Rectal: Occult blood, prostate, testicular or pelvic masses, inguinal lymphadenopathy.

Extremities: >2 cm difference in calf circumference, redness, cyanosis; mottling, tenderness; Homan's sign (tenderness with dorsiflexion of foot); warmth; dilated varicose veins.

Labs: Impedance plethysmography and Doppler studies, venogram; INR/PTT, CBC, electrolytes, BUN, creatinine; ECG, UA, CXR.

Differential Diagnosis: Thrombophlebitis, lymphatic obstruction, cellulitis, muscle injury, hematoma, ruptured Baker's cyst, plantaris rupture, gastrocnemius tear.

CONNECTIVE TISSUE DISEASES

<u>History:</u> Joint pain, fatigue, malaise, weight loss, fever, skin rashes; symmetrical, swelling of upper and lower extremities, morning joint stiffness, photosensitivity, muscle aches and weakness.

Hip and back pain, oral ulcers, weight loss, renal disease; anemia, psychiatric illness, chest pain, dysphagia, heartburn, pleurisy, positional chest pain (pericarditis), Raynaud's syndrome (red, blue or numb hands when exposed to cold); migraine headaches, stroke; depression, hypertension.

<u>Drugs Associated with Lupus:</u> Procainamide, isoniazid, hydralazine, penicillin, sulfonamides, tetracycline, methyldopa (Aldomet).

Physical Exam:

<u>Vitals:</u> Hypertension,

<u>Skin:</u>Skin fibrosis (thickening, scleroderma), calcinosis, telangiectasis, discoid lesions (erythematous plaques), photosensitivity, alopecia, purpura, skin ulcers, rheumatoid nodules, livedo reticularis.

<u>HEENT:</u> Keratoconjunctivitis sicca (dry inflammation of conjunctiva), malar rash (erythematous rash in "butterfly" pattern on face), oral ulcers. Episcleritis/scleritis, xerophthalmia (dry eyes), parotid enlargement.

<u>Chest:</u> Pleural friction rub, fine rale (interstitial fibrosis).

<u>Heart:</u> Cardiac friction rubs, arrhythmias.

<u>Abdomen:</u> Hepatosplenomegaly, abdominal tenderness.

<u>Extremities:</u> Joint deformities, arthralgias, muscle weakness, lymphadenopathy sclerodactyly.

<u>Labs:</u> Electrolytes, creatinine, ANA, LE cell prep, VDRL, ESR, CBC, UA, ECG, complement. UA (proteinuria, casts).

Diagnostic Criteria for Rheumatoid Arthritis: Four or more of the following:

1. Morning stiffness (>6 weeks)
2. Arthritis in 3 or more joints (>6 weeks)
3. Arthritis of hand joints (>6 weeks)
4. Symmetric arthritis (>6 weeks)

5. Rheumatoid nodules

6. Positive rheumatoid factor

7. X-ray abnormalities: Erosions, bony decalcification (especially in hands/wrist).

Diagnostic Criteria for SLE: Four or more of the following;

1. Malar rash

2. Discoid rash

3. Photosensitivity

4. Oral or nasopharyngeal ulcers

5. Nonerosive arthritis

6. Pleuritis/pericarditis

7. Persistent proteinuria

8. Seizures or psychosis

9. Hemolytic anemia

10. Positive lupus erythematosus cell, positive anti-DNA antibody, Sm antibody, false positive VDRL.

11. Positive ANA

PSYCHIATRY

MINI-MENTAL STATUS EXAM

Orientation: What is the year, season, day of week, date, month? - 5 points

What is the state, county, city, hospital, floor ? - 5 points

Registration: Repeat: 3 objects: apple, book, coat. - 3 points

Attention/Calculation: Spell "WORLD" backwards - 5 points

Memory: Recall the names of the previous 3 objects: - 3 points

Language: Name a pencil and a watch - 2 points

Repeat, "No ifs, and's or buts" - 1 point

Three stage command: "Take this paper in your right hand, fold it in half, and
put it on the floor." - 3 points

Written command: "Close your eyes." - 1 point

Write a sentence. - 1 point

Visual Spacial: Copy two overlapping pentagons - 1 point

Total Score 30 Points

Normal: 25-30

Mild intellectual impairment: 20-25

Moderate intellectual impairment: 10-20

Severe intellectual impairment: 0-10

MENTAL STATUS EXAM

1. **Appearance:** Unkept dress, poor hygiene, well groomed.

2. **Mood:** Melancholic, euthymic, euphoric.

3. **Affect:** Congruent, incongruent, blunted.

4. **Form of Thought:** Flight of ideas, circumstantiality, perseveration,
   verbigeration, loosening of associations.

5. **Speech:** Normal, slow, rapid, pressured.

6. **Content of Thoughts:** Appropriate, obsessional, delusion.

7. **Psychomotor Activity:** Alert, agitated, slow.

8. **Insight and Judgement:** Response to hypothetical situations; disorganized, organized.

9. **Cooperation:** Normal, hostile, irritable.

ATTEMPTED SUICIDE
TRICYCLIC ANTIDEPRESSANT OVERDOSE

History: Time suicide was attempted and method. Quantity of pills; motive for attempt. Alcohol intake, other medications; where was medication obtained; possibility of pregnancy, last menstrual period.

Symptoms of TCA Overdose: Dry mouth, hallucinations, seizure, agitation, visual changes.

Psychiatric History: Previous suicide attempts or threats, family support, marital conflict, alcohol or drug abuse. Availability of other dangerous medications or weapons; sources of emotional stress. Precipitating factor for suicide attempt (death, divorce, humiliating event, unemployment, medical illness); further desire to commit suicide; is there a definite plan; was action impulsive or planned.

Detailed account of events 48-hours prior to suicide attempt and events after. Feelings of sadness, guilt, hopelessness, helplessness, persecution. Reasons that a patient has to wish to go on living. Did the patient's believe that he would succeed in suicide. Is the patient upset that he is still alive. Personal or family history of emotional, physical, or sexual abuse.

Family history of depression, suicide, psychiatric disease.

Physical Exam:
General: Level of consciousness, confusion, delirium; anxiety; presence of potentially dangerous objects or substances.

Vitals: BP (hypotension), P (bradycardia), T (hyperpyrexia), R.

HEENT: Signs of trauma; pupil size and reactivity, mydriasis, nystagmus, dry mouth.

Chest: Respiratory pattern, rhonchi (aspiration).

Heart: Rhythm (arrhythmias).

Abdomen: Decreased bowel sounds.

Extremities: Needle marks, wounds; warm, dry skin.

Neuro: Mental status exam; positive Babinski reflexes, tremor, clonus, hyperactive reflexes.

ECG Signs of Antidepressant Overdose: QRS widening, PR or QT interval prolongation, AV block, ventricular tachycardia, Torsades de pointes vertricular arrhythmia.

Labs: Electrolytes, BUN, creatinine, glucose; ABG. Alcohol, acetaminophen levels; CXR, urine toxicology screen.

COMMONLY USED FORMULAS

A-a gradient = $[(P_B - PH_2O) FiO_2 - PCO_2/R] - PO_2$ arterial

= $(713 \times FiO_2 - pCO_2/0.8) - pO_2$ arterial

P_B = 760 mmHg; PH_2O = 47 mmHg ; R ≈ 0.8
normal Aa gradient <10-15 mmHg (room air)

Arterial oxygen capacity = (Hgb(gm)/100 ml) x 1.36 ml O_2/gm Hgb

Arterial O_2 content = 1.36(Hgb)(SaO2)+0.003(PaO2)= NL 20 vol%

O_2 delivery = CO x arterial O_2 content = NL 640-1000 ml O_2/min

Cardiac output = HR x stroke volume

CO L/min = $\dfrac{125 \text{ ml } O_2/\text{min}/M^2}{8.5\{(1.36)(Hgb)(SaO2) - (1.36)(Hgb)(SvO2)\}}$ x 100

(need to multiply by M^2 to get CO estimate for a patient. This is CI estimate)

Note: 125 is a crude estimate for normals
Normal CO = 4-6 L/min

SVR = $\dfrac{MAP - CVP}{CO_{L/min}}$ x 80 = NL 800-1200 dyne/sec/cm^2

PVR = $\dfrac{PA - PCWP}{CO_{L/min}}$ x 80 = NL 45-120 dyne/sec/cm^2

GFR ml/min = $\dfrac{(140 - age) \times wt \text{ in Kg}}{72 \text{ (males)} \times \text{serum Cr (mg/dl)}}$
           85 (females) x serum Cr (mg/dl)

Creatinine clearance = $\dfrac{U \text{ Cr (mg/100 mL)} \times U \text{ vol (mL)}}{P \text{ Cr (mg/100 mL)} \times time \text{ (1440 min for 24h)}}$

Normal creatinine clearance = 100-125 ml/min(males), 85-105(females)

Body water deficit (L) = $\dfrac{0.6(\text{weight kg})([\text{measured serum Na}]-140)}{140}$

Osmolality mOsm/kg = 2[Na+ K] + $\dfrac{BUN}{2.8}$ + $\dfrac{glucose}{18}$ = NL 270-290 $\dfrac{mOsm}{kg}$

Fractional excreted Na = $\dfrac{U \text{ Na}/ \text{Serum Na}}{U \text{ Cr}/ \text{Serum Cr}}$ x 100 = NL<1%

Anion Gap = Na + K - (Cl + HCO3)

For each 100 mg/dl ↑ in glucose, Na+ ↓ by 1.6 mEq/L.

Corrected
serum Ca^+ (mg/dl) = measured Ca mg/dl + 0.8 x (4 - albumin g/dl)

Ideal body weight males = 50 kg for first 5 feet of height + 2.3 kg for each additional inch.

Ideal body weight females = 45.5 kg for first 5 feet + 2.3 kg for each additional inch.

Basal energy expenditure (BEE):
  Males=66 + (13.7 x actual weight Kg) + (5 x height cm)-(6.8 x age)
  Females= 655+(9.6 x actual weight Kg)+(1.7 x height cm)-(4.7 x age)

Nitrogen Balance = Gm protein intake/6.25 - urine urea nitrogen - (3-4 gm/d insensible loss)

Predicted Maximal Heart Rate = 220 - age

Normal ECG Intervals (sec)
PR	0.12-0.20
QRS	0.06-0.08

Heart rate/min	**Q-T**
60	0.33-0.43
70	0.31-0.41
80	0.29-0.38
90	0.28-0.36
100	0.27-0.35

DRUG LEVELS OF COMMON MEDICATIONS

DRUG	THERAPEUTIC RANGE*
Amikacin	Peak 25-30; trough <10 mcg/ml
Amitriptyline	100-250 ng/ml
Carbamazepine	4-10 mcg/ml
Chloramphenicol	Peak 10-15; trough <5 mcg/ml
Desipramine	150-300 ng/ml
Digitoxin	10-30 ng/ml
Digoxin	0.8-2.0 ng/ml
Disopyramide	2-5 mcg/ml
Doxepin	75-200 ng/ml
Ethosuximide	40-100 mcg/ml
Flecainide	0.2-1.0 mcg/ml
Gentamicin	Peak 6.0-8.0; trough <2.0 mcg/ml
Imipramine	150-300 ng/ml
Lidocaine	2-5 mcg/ml
Lithium	0.5-1.4 meq/L
Nortriptyline	50-150 ng/ml
Phenobarbital	10-30 meq/ml
Phenytoin**	8-20 mcg/ml
Procainamide	4.0-8.0 mcg/ml
Quinidine	2.5-5.0 mcg/ml
Salicylate	15-25 mg/dl
Streptomycin	Peak 10-20; trough <5 mcg/ml
Theophylline	8-20 mcg/ml
Tocainide	4-10 mcg/ml
Valproic acid	50-100 mcg/ml
Vancomycin	Peak 30-40; trough <10 mcg/ml

* The therapeutic range of some drugs may vary depending on the reference lab used.

** Therapeutic range of phenytoin is 4-10 mcg/ml in presence of significant azotemia and/or hypoalbuminemia.

COMMONLY USED ABBREVIATIONS

1/2NS	0.45% saline solution	CSF	cerebrospinal fluid
a.c.	ante cibum (before meals)	CT	computerized tomography
ABG	arterial blood gas		
ac	before meals	CVA	cerebrovascular accident
ACTH	adrenocorticotropic hormone		
ad	right ear	CVP	central venous pressure
ad lib	ad libitum (as needed or desired)		
		CXR	chest x-ray
ADH	antidiuretic hormone	d/c	discharge; discontinue
AFB	acid-fast bacillus		
alk phos	alkaline phosphatase	D5W	5% dextrose water solution; also D10W, D50W
ALT	alanine aminotransferase		
am	morning		
AMA.	against medical advice	DIC	disseminated intravascular coagulation
amp	ampule		
amt	amount	diff	differential count
AMV	assisted mandatory ventilation; assist mode ventilation	dil	dilute
		DKA	diabetic ketoacidosis
		dL	deciliter
ANA	antinuclear antibody	DOSS	docusate sodium sulfosuccinate--a stool softener
ante	before		
AP	anteroposterior		
aq	water		
ARDS	adult respiratory distress syndrome	DT's	delirium tremens
		ECG	electrocardiogram
as, al	left ear	ER	emergency room
ASA	acetylsalicylic acid	ERCP	endoscopic retrograde cholangiopancreatography
AST	aspartate aminotransferase		
au	both ears		
bid	bis in die (twice a day)		
B-12	vitamin B-12 (cyanocobalamin)	ESR	erythrocyte sedimentation rate
		ET	endotracheal tube
BM	bowel movement	ETOH	alcohol
BP	blood pressure	F	Fahrenheit
BUN	blood urea nitrogen	Fe/TIBC	iron/total iron-binding capacity
c/o	complaint of		
c̄	cum (with)		
C and S	culture and sensitivity	Fe	iron
C	centigrade	FEV$_1$	forced expiratory volume (in one second)
C3, C4	third and fourth complement components		
		FiO2	fractional inspired oxygen
Ca	calcium		
cap	capsule	fl	fluid
CBC	complete blood count; includes hemoglobin, hematocrit, red blood cell indices, white blood cell count, and platelets	g	gram(s)
		GC	gonococcal; gonococcus
		GFR	glomerular filtration rate
cc	cubic centimeter		
CCU	coronary care unit	GI	gastrointestinal
cm	centimeter	gm	gram
CMF	cyclophosphamide, methotrexate, and fluorouracil	gt	drop
		gtt	drops
CNS	central nervous system	h .hr	hour
CO$_2$	carbon dioxide	H20	water
COPD	chronic obstructive pulmonary disease	HBsAG	hepatitis B surface antigen
		HCO3	bicarbonate
CPK	creatinine phosphokinase	Hct	hematocrit
CPK-MB	myocardial-specific CPK isoenzyme	HDL	high-density lipoprotein
CPR	cardiopulmonary resuscitation		

Hg	mercury		(insulin)
Hgb	hemoglobin concentration	NPO	nulla per os (nothing by mouth)
HIV	human immunodeficiency virus	NS	normal saline solution (0.9%)
hr	hour	NSAID	nonsteroidal anti-inflammatory drug
hs	hora somni (bedtime, hour of sleep)	O2	oxygen
IM	intramuscular	OD	right eye
I & O	intake and output--measurement of the patient's intake by any route (mouth, intravenous, rectum) and output by any route, including urine, vomit, diarrhea, and fluid from bleeding or drainage	oint	ointment
		OS	left eye
		Osm	osmolality
		OT	occupational therapy
		OTC	over the counter
IU	international units	OU	each eye
ICU	intensive care unit	oz	ounce
IgM	immunoglobulin M	p, post	after
IMV	intermittent mandatory ventilation	p.c.	post cibum (after meals)
INH	isoniazid	PA	posteroanterior; pulmonary artery
IPPB	intermittent positive-pressure breathing	PaO2	arterial oxygen pressure
IV	intravenous or intravenously	pAO2	partial pressure of oxygen in alveolar gas
IVP	intravenous pyelogram; intravenous piggyback		
		PB	phenobarbital
K, K+	potassium	pc	after meals
kcal	kilocalorie	pCO2	partial pressure of carbon dioxide
KCL	potassium chloride		
KPO4	potassium phosphate	PEEP	positive end-expiratory pressure
KUB	x-ray of abdomen (kidneys, ureters, bowels)		
		per	by
L	liter	pH	hydrogen ion concentration (H +)
LDH	lactate dehydrogenase		
LDL	low-density lipoprotein	PID	pelvic inflammatory disease
liq	liquid		
LLQ	left lower quadrant	pm	afternoon
LP	lumbar puncture, low potency	PO	orally
		PO	per os (by mouth)
LR	lactated Ringer's (solution)	pO2	partial pressure of oxygen
MB	myocardial band		
MBC	minimal bacterial concentration	polys	polymorphonuclear leukocytes
mcg	microgram	PPD	purified protein derivative
mEq	milliequivalent		
mg	milligram	PR	per rectum
Mg	magnesium	prn	as needed
Mg	magnesium	prn	pro re nata (as needed)
MgSO4	Magnesium Sulfate		
MI	myocardial infarction	Pro	prothrombin
MIC	minimum inhibitory concentration	PT	physical therapy; prothrombin time
mL	milliliter	PTCA	percutaneous transluminal coronary angioplasty
mm	millimeter		
MOM	Milk of Magnesia		
MRI	magnetic resonance imaging	PTT	partial thromboplastin time
Na	sodium		
NaHCO3	sodium bicarbonate	PVC	premature ventricular contraction
Neuro	neurologic		
NG	nasogastric	q	quaque (every)
NKA	no known allergies		
NPH	neutral protamine Hagedorn		

	q6h, q2h	every 6 hours; every 2 hours	
qid	quarter in die (four times a day)		
qAM	every morning		
qd	quaque die (every day)		
qh	every hour		
qhs	every night before bedtime		
qid	4 times a day		
qOD	every other day		
qs	quantity sufficient		
R/O	rule out		
RA	rheumatoid arthritis; room air; right atrial		
Resp	respiratory rate		
RL	Ringer's lactated solution (also LR)		
ROM	range of motion		
rt.	right		
s	sine (without)		
s/p	status post (the condition of being after)		
sat	saturated		
SBP	systolic blood pressure		
SC	subcutaneously		
SGOT	serum glutamic-oxaloacetic transaminase (AST)		
SGPT	serum glutamic-pyruvic transaminase (ALT)		
SIADH	syndrome of inappropriate antidiuretic hormone		
SL	sublingually under tongue		
SLE	systemic lupus erythematosus		
SMA-12	sequential multiple analysis; a panel of 12 chemistry tests performed together on a 12-channel autoanalyzer. Tests generally include Na^+, K^+, HCO3 , Chloride , BUN, glucose, creatinine, bilirubin, calcium, total protein, albumin, and alkaline phosphatase. Other chemistry panels include SMA-6 and SMA-20		
SMX	sulfamethoxazole		
sob	shortness of breath		
sol	solution		
SQ	under the skin		
ss	one-half		
STAT	statim (immediately)		
susp	suspension		
t.i.d.	ter in die (three times a day)		
T4	thyroxine level (T4)		
tab	tablet		
TB	tuberculosis		
Tbsp	tablespoon		
Temp	temperature		
TIA	transient ischemic attack		
tid	three times a day		
TKO	to keep open, an infusion rate (usually 500 mL/24h)--		

		just enough to keep the IV from clotting
TMP	trimethoprim	
TMP-SMX	trimethoprim-sulfamethoxazole combination	
TPA	tissue plasminogen activator	
TSH	thyroid-stimulating hormone	
tsp	teaspoon	
U	units	
UA	urinalysis	
ung	ointment	
URI	upper respiratory infection	
USP	United States Pharmacopeia	
Ut Dict	as directed	
UTI	urinary tract infection	
VAC	vincristine, Adriamycin, and cyclophosphamide	
vag	vaginal	
VC	vital capacity	
VDRL	Venereal Disease Research Laboratory	
VF	ventricular function	
V fib	ventricular fibrillation	
VLDL	very low-density lipoprotein	
Vol	volume	
VS	vital signs	
VT	ventricular tachycardia	
W	water	
WBC	white blood count	
x	times	

INDEX

ORDER FORM

Books from Current Clinical Strategies Publishing:

Current Clinical Strategies, Practice Parameters in Medicine, Primary Care, Family Practice, and Gynecology	#___ x	$16.75
Current Clinical Strategies, **PEDIATRIC** DRUG RESOURCE	#___ x	$8.75
Handbook of Anesthesiology Mark Ezekiel, MD	#___ x	$8.75
Manual of HIV/AIDS Therapy Laurence Peiperl, MD	#___ x	$8.75
Current Clinical Strategies, MEDICINE, Paul D. Chan, MD NEW 1994 edition	#___ x	$8.75
Current Clinical Strategies, GYNECOLOGY & OBSTETRICS, NEW 1995 edition	#___ x	$10.75
Current Clinical Strategies, PEDIATRICS, NEW 1995 edition	#___ x	$8.75
FAMILY MEDICINE, NEW 1995 edition Pediatrics, Medicine, Gynecology, Obstetrics	#___ x	$26.25
DIAGNOSTIC HISTORY & PHYSICAL EXAMINATION in MEDICINE	#___ x	$8.75
OUTPATIENT MEDICINE	#___ x	$8.75
CRITICAL CARE MEDICINE, 1995 edition	#___ x	$12.75
PSYCHIATRY	#___ x	$8.75
HANDBOOK OF PSYCHIATRIC DRUG THERAPY	#___ x	$8.75
Current Clinical Strategies, SURGERY	#___ x	$8.75
Current Clinical Strategies, PHYSICIAN'S DRUG RESOURCE (Adult dosages)	#___ x	$8.75

Shipping and Handling, add $2.00 per book $ _____

                                        Total $ _____

Enclose the cover of your old edition, and receive $2.00 off your order when you purchase the new edition.

Please complete reverse side.

Prices are in US dollars. Other countries, send equivalent amount in foreign check. Prices and Availability subject to change without notice.

Order by Phone: 714-965-9400 (a bill will be sent with order)

Order by Mail. Send order & check payable to:

Current Clinical Strategies Publishing
9550 Warner Ave, Suite 213
Fountain Valley, Ca USA 92708-2822

Return Address: _____

_____

_____

_____

Phone Number: (_____)_____

Comments:

We appreciate your comments about our books and software.

Suggested additions, problems or criticisms:

_____

_____

_____

_____

_____

_____

_____

ORDER FORM

Books from Current Clinical Strategies Publishing:

Current Clinical Strategies, Practice Parameters in Medicine, Primary Care, Family Practice, and Gynecology	#___ x	$16.75
Current Clinical Strategies, **PEDIATRIC** DRUG RESOURCE	#___ x	$8.75
Handbook of Anesthesiology Mark Ezekiel, MD	#___ x	$8.75
Manual of HIV/AIDS Therapy Laurence Peiperl, MD	#___ x	$8.75
Current Clinical Strategies, MEDICINE, Paul D. Chan, MD NEW 1994 edition	#___ x	$8.75
Current Clinical Strategies, GYNECOLOGY & OBSTETRICS, NEW 1995 edition	#___ x	$10.75
Current Clinical Strategies, PEDIATRICS, NEW 1995 edition	#___ x	$8.75
FAMILY MEDICINE, NEW 1995 edition Pediatrics, Medicine, Gynecology, Obstetrics	#___ x	$26.25
DIAGNOSTIC HISTORY & PHYSICAL EXAMINATION in MEDICINE	#___ x	$8.75
OUTPATIENT MEDICINE	#___ x	$8.75
CRITICAL CARE MEDICINE, 1995 edition	#___ x	$12.75
PSYCHIATRY	#___ x	$8.75
HANDBOOK OF PSYCHIATRIC DRUG THERAPY	#___ x	$8.75
Current Clinical Strategies, SURGERY	#___ x	$8.75
Current Clinical Strategies, PHYSICIAN'S DRUG RESOURCE (Adult dosages)	#___ x	$8.75

Shipping and Handling, add $2.00 per book $ _____

Total $ _____

Enclose the cover of your old edition, and receive $2.00 off your order when you purchase the new edition.

Please complete reverse side.

Prices are in US dollars. Other countries, send equivalent amount in foreign check. Prices and Availability subject to change without notice.

Order by Phone: 714-965-9400 (a bill will be sent with order)

Order by Mail. Send order & check payable to:

Current Clinical Strategies Publishing
9550 Warner Ave, Suite 213
Fountain Valley, Ca USA 92708-2822

Return Address: _____

_____

_____

_____

Phone Number: (_____)_____

Comments:

We appreciate your comments about our books and software.

Suggested additions, problems or criticisms:

_____

_____

_____

_____

_____

_____

_____

ORDER FORM

Books from Current Clinical Strategies Publishing:

Current Clinical Strategies, Practice Parameters in Medicine, Primary Care, Family Practice, and Gynecology	#___ x	$16.75
Current Clinical Strategies, **PEDIATRIC** DRUG RESOURCE	#___ x	$8.75
Handbook of Anesthesiology Mark Ezekiel, MD	#___ x	$8.75
Manual of HIV/AIDS Therapy Laurence Peiperl, MD	#___ x	$8.75
Current Clinical Strategies, MEDICINE, Paul D. Chan, MD NEW 1994 edition	#___ x	$8.75
Current Clinical Strategies, GYNECOLOGY & OBSTETRICS, NEW 1995 edition	#___ x	$10.75
Current Clinical Strategies, PEDIATRICS, NEW 1995 edition	#___ x	$8.75
FAMILY MEDICINE, NEW 1995 edition Pediatrics, Medicine, Gynecology, Obstetrics	#___ x	$26.25
DIAGNOSTIC HISTORY & PHYSICAL EXAMINATION in MEDICINE	#___ x	$8.75
OUTPATIENT MEDICINE	#___ x	$8.75
CRITICAL CARE MEDICINE, 1995 edition	#___ x	$12.75
PSYCHIATRY	#___ x	$8.75
HANDBOOK OF PSYCHIATRIC DRUG THERAPY	#___ x	$8.75
Current Clinical Strategies, SURGERY	#___ x	$8.75
Current Clinical Strategies, PHYSICIAN'S DRUG RESOURCE (Adult dosages)	#___ x	$8.75

Shipping and Handling, add $2.00 per book $ _____

Total $ _____

Enclose the cover of your old edition, and receive $2.00 off your order when you purchase the new edition.

Please complete reverse side.

Prices are in US dollars. Other countries, send equivalent amount in foreign check. Prices and Availability subject to change without notice.

Order by Phone: 714-965-9400 (a bill will be sent with order)

Order by Mail. Send order & check payable to:

Current Clinical Strategies Publishing
9550 Warner Ave, Suite 213
Fountain Valley, Ca USA 92708-2822

Return Address: _____

_____

_____

_____

Phone Number: (_____)_____

Comments:

We appreciate your comments about our books and software.

Suggested additions, problems or criticisms:

_____

_____

_____

_____

_____

_____

_____

_____